SpringerBriefs in Statistics

JSS Research Series in Statistics

The current research of statistics in Japan has expanded in several directions in line with recent trends in academic activities in the area of statistics and statistical sciences over the globe. The core of these research activities in statistics in Japan has been the Japan Statistical Society (JSS). This society, the oldest and largest academic organization for statistics in Japan, was founded in 1931 by a handful of pioneer statisticians and economists and now has a history of about 80 years. Many distinguished scholars have been members, including the influential statistician Hirotugu Akaike, who was a past president of JSS, and the notable mathematician Kiyosi Itô, who was an earlier member of the Institute of Statistical Mathematics (ISM), which has been a closely related organization since the establishment of ISM. The society has two academic journals: the Journal of the Japan Statistical Society (English Series) and the Journal of the Japan Statistical Society (Japanese Series). The membership of JSS consists of researchers, teachers, and professional statisticians in many different fields including mathematics, statistics, engineering, medical sciences, government statistics, economics, business, psychology, education, and many other natural, biological, and social sciences. The JSS Series of Statistics aims to publish recent results of current research activities in the areas of statistics and statistical sciences in Japan that otherwise would not be available in English; they are complementary to the two JSS academic journals, both English and Japanese. Because the scope of a research paper in academic journals inevitably has become narrowly focused and condensed in recent years, this series is intended to fill the gap between academic research activities and the form of a single academic paper. The series will be of great interest to a wide audience of researchers, teachers, professional statisticians, and graduate students in many countries who are interested in statistics and statistical sciences, in statistical theory, and in various areas of statistical applications.

More information about this series at http://www.springer.com/series/13497

Takashi Daimon · Akihiro Hirakawa ·
Shigeyuki Matsui

Dose-Finding Designs for Early-Phase Cancer Clinical Trials

A Brief Guidebook to Theory and Practice

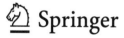 Springer

Takashi Daimon
Department of Biostatistics
Hyogo College of Medicine
Nishinomiya, Hyogo, Japan

Shigeyuki Matsui
Graduate School of Medicine
Nagoya University
Nagoya, Aichi, Japan

Akihiro Hirakawa
Department of Biostatistics and
Bioinformatics, Graduate School of
Medicine
The University of Tokyo
Tokyo, Japan

ISSN 2191-544X   ISSN 2191-5458   (electronic)
SpringerBriefs in Statistics
ISSN 2364-0057   ISSN 2364-0065   (electronic)
JSS Research Series in Statistics
ISBN 978-4-431-55584-1   ISBN 978-4-431-55585-8   (eBook)
https://doi.org/10.1007/978-4-431-55585-8

This Springer imprint is published by the registered company Springer Japan KK part of Springer Nature.
The registered company address is: Shiroyama Trust Tower, 4-3-1 Toranomon, Minato-ku, Tokyo
105-6005, Japan

To our beloved families and our dear ex-colleagues/colleagues at Hyogo College of Medicine, the University of Tokyo, and Nagoya University.

Preface

The key to successful anticancer drug treatment is determination of the optimal dose to be administered to the patient. The optimal dose is conventionally identified by conducting a phase I trial of a new agent, in which the relationship between the dose and toxicity is primarily investigated; hence, the maximum tolerated dose (MTD) or phase II recommended dose is determined. The most commonly used phase I trial design is the so-called "3 + 3 design." However, the statistical community has repeatedly demonstrated that this design is not optimal with regard to both MTD determination and the chance of MTD allocation to trial participants. Consequently, many dose-finding designs have been developed to replace the 3 + 3 design. The aim of the present book is to provide a comprehensive introduction to these designs.

This book is intended to serve as a brief handbook for graduate students and practitioners of biostatistics, as well as for clinical investigators involved in the design, implementation, monitoring, and analysis of dose-finding trials, so as to choose the best dose-finding designs for early-phase cancer clinical trials. An overview of advanced topics and discussions relevant to this field is also provided, for the benefit of researchers in biostatistics and statistical science.

This book begins by introducing background information and fundamental concepts regarding dose-finding in early-phase clinical trials, and then presents both traditional and recently developed dose-finding designs for phase I trials targeting toxicity outcome evaluation. These designs include rule-based designs, e.g., the most frequently used 3 + 3 designs; model-based designs including the standard-bearer, namely, the continual reassessment method (CRM); and model-assisted designs, e.g., Bayesian optimal interval (BOIN) designs. In addition, related topics and more complex designs are presented. Dose-finding designs considering both toxicity and efficacy outcomes are also discussed. Finally, this book elucidates the topic of immunotherapy, which has gained considerable attention as a cancer treatment option, and introduces several early-phase dose-finding designs for immunotherapeutic agent trials.

In detail, the main text of this book is organized as follows. Chapter 1 overviews the clinical research and development process of anticancer drugs, describes the basic concept of early-phase trials, and outlines dose-finding designs for early-phase trials. Chapter 2 focuses on rule-based designs considering toxicity alone. The most commonly used $3 + 3$ design receives particular attention here, and it is emphasized that this approach poorly identifies the MTD despite its simplicity and transparency. Then, an overview of alternative rule-based designs that can improve upon the performance of the $3 + 3$ design is presented, along with a discussion of related topics. Chapter 3 provides a detailed description of the concepts, theories, properties, advantages, and disadvantages of the CRM, and also overviews related or extended model-based designs considering toxicity alone, along with more complex designs. Chapter 4 describes model-assisted designs considering toxicity alone, including the modified toxicity probability interval (mTPI) design and its improved version (the mTPI-2 design), the keyboard design, and the BOIN design. Again, related topics are also discussed. Chapter 5 outlines dose-finding designs considering both efficacy and toxicity, classifying them into rule-based, model-based, and model-assisted designs. Finally, Chap. 6 introduces dose-finding designs for early-phase immunotherapy trials and discusses the topic of dose expansion cohorts.

The authors are grateful for the support of a Grant-in-Aid for Scientific Research (Nos. 15K00058, 15K15948, 16H06299, and 17K00045) from the Ministry of Education, Culture, Sports, Science, and Technology of Japan for this book project.

Hyogo, Japan   Takashi Daimon
March 2019   Akihiro Hirakawa
                                                                                 Shigeyuki Matsui

Contents

Acronyms

AUC	Area under the curve
BOIN	Bayesian optimal interval
CA	Chemotherapeutic agent
CRM	Continual reassessment method
DLT	Dose-limiting toxicity
EWOC	Escalation with overdose control
IA	Immunotherapeutic agent
MTA	Molecularly targeted agent
MTD	Maximum tolerated dose
mTPI	Modified toxicity probability interval
MTS	Maximum tolerated schedule
NCI-CTCAE	National Cancer Institute Common Terminology Criteria for Adverse Events
OD	Optimal dose
RP2D	Recommended phase II dose

Chapter 1
Early-Phase Cancer Clinical Trials

Abstract The primary objective of early-phase (phase I, or phase I/II) clinical trials of a given anticancer agent is to determine its optimal dose (OD) to be administered to a cancer patient, so as to obtain the highest efficacy while maintaining admissible toxicity. Thus, in oncology, early-phase trials for anticancer agents are also called "dose-finding" trials. For a chemotherapeutic or cytotoxic agent, classically, the OD is determined in the phase I trial, in which toxicity alone is primarily evaluated. Here, the highest tested safe dose with tolerable toxicity, called the "maximum tolerated dose (MTD)," is determined. This approach is adopted because monotonic increases in both toxicity and efficacy with increasing dose are assumed; thus, the MTD corresponds to the recommended phase II dose, and is also expected to yield the highest efficacy among the tested doses. However, this reasoning may not hold for molecularly targeted or cytostatic agents, or for immunotherapeutic agents (IAs). The ODs of such agents are found in phase I/II trials, in which both toxicity and efficacy are evaluated to determine the dose that yields the highest efficacy and admissible toxicity, or the dose that also yields the required immune response (particularly for IAs). This distinction exists because the efficacy does not always monotonically increase with a higher dose, even if the toxicity increases in this manner. In this chapter, we overview the clinical research and development process of anticancer drugs, describe the basic concepts of early-phase trials, and outline various dose-finding designs for early-phase trials.

Keywords Oncology · Optimal dose · Chemotherapy · Molecularly targeted therapy · Immunotherapy

1.1 Cancer Clinical Trials

Clinical trials are conducted to evaluate new medical interventions; thus, they constitute the basis of evidence-based medicine by answering clinical questions on the safety and effectiveness of novel interventions that may yield improvements in clinical practice. Usually, if a certain new medical intervention is based on a new agent, the related clinical research and development includes clinical trials consisting of multiple phases: phase I, II, and III trials. Phase I trials are conducted as the first trials of any new agent in humans (i.e., healthy volunteers or patients presenting life-threatening diseases such as AIDS or cancer), so as to evaluate its short-term safety and efficacy. Phase II trials are conducted after the phase I trials and involve patients with a particular disease; hence, the relatively long-term efficacy and safety of the agent are evaluated. The larger phase III trials follow the phase II trials and are intended to confirm the efficacy and safety of the target agent through comparison with the existing best-available therapy. Phase III trials are often conducted to obtain approval for use of the target agent as a drug (see, e.g., Yin 2012). In some cases, phase IV trials are conducted after this approval has been attained, so as to gain additional information on the risks and benefits of the drug.

In principle, this process is valid for clinical research and development of cancer treatments, particularly those involving anticancer drugs. However, there are many types of cancer treatment: surgical therapy, radiotherapy, chemotherapy, targeted therapy, immunotherapy, hormonal therapy, and so on (see, e.g., Green et al. 2003; Ting 2006; Crowley and Hoering 2012). Conventionally, phase I trials are conducted to evaluate the safety, tolerability, and pharmacokinetics of an investigational drug in humans (usually cancer patients) for the first time, based on dose-finding studies involving a limited number of patients (usually no more than tens of patients). Hence, the highest safe dose with tolerable toxicity, i.e., the maximum tolerated dose (MTD), is determined, along with the recommended phase II dose (RP2D). Phase II trials are then conducted to evaluate the efficacy of the investigational drug by observing the tumor response or the progression-free or overall survival (in cases where observation of the tumor response is particularly difficult or unreliable). These trials are based on single- or multi-arm studies involving a larger number of patients than those included in the dose-finding studies. Hence, the merit of testing the investigational drug further for antitumor activity is decided. Finally, phase III trials are conducted to compare the investigational drug with a standard treatment by observing the overall survival or, in some cases, progression-free survival, for quite a large number of patients. These trials are usually implemented as head-to-head comparative studies, in which the superiority or, sometimes, the inferiority of the investigational drug to the standard treatment is confirmed. In this book, we focus on early-phase trials only, including phase I and phase I/II trials, for anticancer agents oriented toward chemotherapy, targeted therapy, and immunotherapy in oncology.

1.2 Basic Concept of Early-Phase Trials

Anticancer agents present a risk of frequent and serious adverse events due to their high toxicity; however, their therapeutic effects may benefit cancer patients, e.g., through tumor size reduction or provision of prolonged progression-free or overall survival (see, e.g., Horstmann et al. 2005; Kurzrock and Benjamin 2005). The individual patients adopted as subjects in early-phase trials usually present advanced cases for which extended life expectancy cannot be achieved or have symptoms that cannot be alleviated via standard therapies; thus, they are prepared to accept the benefits of the anticancer agent regardless of the toxicity risks (see, e.g., Daugherty et al. 1995; Tomamichel et al. 2000; Cohen et al. 2001). Consequently, early-phase trials are designed to minimize the likelihood of treating patients with unsafe or ineffective doses, while balancing risk and benefit, within a limited maximum sample size of tens of to one hundred patients. To correct an initial, incorrect guess at the dose–toxicity and dose–efficacy relationship, the dose must be immediately escalated if the observed toxicity or efficacy is low, but immediately de-escalated if the observed toxicity is unacceptably high (see, e.g., O'Quigley and Chevret 1991; Eisenhauer et al. 2000; Paoletti et al. 2006). Thus, the aim is to treat the patients included in the trial at the dose having the highest efficacy with admissible toxicity. The early-phase trial for an agent in oncology is, thus, considered to be the "dose-finding" trial, and finds the MTD or the dose having the highest efficacy with admissible toxicity, of the agent.

1.2.1 Early-Phase Trials for Chemotherapeutic Agents

Anticancer agents for chemotherapy, namely, chemotherapeutic agents (CAs), target the cell division process, following the rationale that cancer cells are more likely to be actively replicating than normal cells because of their mechanisms of action. Unfortunately, as CA actions are not specific, these agents kill both fast-growing cancer cells and normal cells that grow and divide quickly. In this sense, CAs are cytotoxic, and are also called "cytotoxic agents." Classically, the primary objective of a phase I trial for a cytotoxic agent is to estimate the MTD of the agent and to determine the RP2D. The secondary objectives include a pharmacokinetic (and, if possible, pharmacodynamic) evaluation, along with observation of the effects of the agent-based treatment.

From a safety perspective, the MTD can be regarded as the upper limit for the admissible dose, and is determined from both data on the doses used to treat patients participating in the phase I trials and information on the presence or absence of dose-limiting toxicity (DLT) at those doses. Thus, the doses administered in phase I trials are candidates for the MTD. They are generally fixed at multiple and discrete doses; thus, they are often referred to as "dose levels"; this is similar to the term "levels of a factor" in experiment design. Further, the dose evaluated at one dose level lower than the MTD is often considered to be the RP2D. The DLT is defined as that at which unacceptable adverse effects are encountered, which force treatment termination or continuation at a reduced dose. In the field of oncology, adverse effects are evaluated based on the National Cancer Institute Common Terminology Criteria for Adverse Events (NCI-CTCAE) with the following grades: none–mild (grades 0–1), moderate (grade 2), dose-limiting (grade 3), and unacceptable (grades 4–5). The unacceptable adverse effects that constitute DLTs are decided for each agent by a group of clinical investigators. DLTs can include hematologic toxicity, such as neutropenia persisting for a prespecified period, febrile neutropenia, thrombocytopenia, and anemia;

and non-hematologic toxicity, such as nausea, vomiting, diarrhea, and liver function abnormality. Unless specifically noted, the DLT is simply referred to as "toxicity" in this book, so as to conform to the conventional terminology used in most of the cited research papers.

Note that the definition of the MTD can differ among trials and clinicians (Storer 1989); however, it can be qualitatively defined as the largest dose at which the patient can tolerate the resulting toxicity. Quantitatively, the MTD is defined as the dose at which the probability of toxicity for the patient cohort of the trial is close to a certain acceptable target value, with consideration of the tolerance distribution in the true relationship between the dose and toxic response (which is, of course, unknown) (Storer 1989). Generally, this acceptable value is set to approximately 0.2–0.33; hereinafter, this value is referred to as the "target toxicity probability level." In particular, when a cytotoxic agent targets intracellular DNA or acts on organelles to kill cancer cells, dose escalation is expected to increase the chances of both a toxic response and a therapeutic effect. Therefore, the MTD is considered to be the only clinically appropriate dose having the capacity to impart a certain therapeutic effect while maintaining safety.

In some cases, to investigate whether a certain dose produces notable efficacy, a so-called phase I/II trial is planned, which combines phase I and II trials into one trial (Yan et al. 2018). There are two approaches toward combining these two trial types. One approach involves implementation of the phase I trial seamlessly followed by the phase II trial. In this approach, the agent toxicity is evaluated and doses with admissible toxicity are identified for patients enrolled in the phase I component; then, the agent efficacy is evaluated using the MTD, RP2D, or several doses with admissible toxicity for the patients enrolled in the phase II component (note that these patients could differ from those in the phase I component). Another approach involves simultaneous implementation of both phase I and II components for a prespecified number of enrolled patients, in which the toxicity and efficacy are simultaneously evaluated. However, regardless of the specific approach, the primary objective is to determine the dose having the highest efficacy with admissible toxicity.

1.2.2   Early-Phase Trials for Molecularly Targeted Agents

Molecularly targeted therapy is a type of cancer treatment that blocks the growth, division, and spread of cancer cells. Most molecularly targeted therapies are based on either small-molecule agents or monoclonal antibody agents. The former can enter cells easily, but the latter cannot. Consequently, small-molecule agents are used for targets within cells, whereas monoclonal antibody agents act on specific targets on the outer surfaces of cancer cells. Note that administration of monoclonal antibodies is also considered a type of immunotherapy, because these antibodies aid the immune system in cancer cell destruction. As a consequence, molecularly targeted agents (MTAs) have different toxicity profiles to CAs. In fact, a survey by Paoletti et al. (2014) suggests that a longer toxicity assessment period beyond cycle 1 is needed to decide the RP2D for MTAs, and that specific grade-2 toxicities should be incorporated into the DLT definitions. In addition, different from the behavior of CAs, MTA efficacy may not increase with dose; specifically, increase for lower doses and then reach a plateau, or possibly decrease for higher doses. Therefore, considering these differences between MTAs and CAs, conventional phase I trials for CAs that rely on the MTD-based approach to identify the RP2D may not be suitable for MTAs. Thus, phase I or I/II trials considering both toxicity and efficacy are recommended for MTA dose optimization (Yan et al. 2018).

1.2.3 Early-Phase Trials for Immunotherapeutic Agents

Recently, immunotherapy, which is a type of cancer treatment that helps the human immune system target cancer directly, has attracted considerable attention as a cancer treatment option (Couzin-Frankel 2013). Because the immune system recognizes and attacks a tumor in this approach, immunotherapy is more personalized than molecularly targeted therapies. The various types of immunotherapy include treatments involving checkpoint inhibitors, adaptive cell transfer, monoclonal antibodies, vaccines, and cytokines. Clinical research and development procedures for immunotherapeutic agents (IAs) targeting the various types of immunotherapy are rapidly evolving. However, as for MTAs, conventional phase I trials for CAs may not be suitable for IAs. One reason for this lack of suitability is that an MTD may not be identifiable for IAs. In fact, Morrissey et al. (2016) have shown that, in single-agent phase I trials of nivolmub, pembrolizumab, and iplimumab, an MTD cannot be identified. This issue commonly arises in phase I trials of cancer vaccines because of their flat dose–toxicity relationship. It should also be noted that toxic profiles are different between the aforementioned checkpoint infibitors (see, e.g., Postel-Vinay et al. 2016) and vaccines (see, e.g., Wang et al. 2018). In addition, the assumption of a monotonic increases in efficacy with increasing dose may not be appropriate for IAs, because the immunotherapy mechanism of action is based on boosting of the immune system. Therefore, phase I/II trial designs considering toxicity, efficacy, and immune response are recommended for IA dose optimization.

1.3 Dose-Finding Designs for Early-Phase Clinical Trials

Numerous dose-finding designs for phase I trials that primarily evaluate toxicity alone have been proposed, so as to overcome the problems encountered in practice while acknowledging the needs of clinicians (as examples of original research, see O'Quigley and Chevret 1991; Rosenberger and Haines 2002; Potter 2006; as examples of books on this topic, see Chevret 2006; Ting 2006; Berry et al. 2010; Crowley and Hoering 2012; O'Quigley et al. 2017). These designs differ in their use of the data on the toxicity induced by the doses administered during trials. However, during a trial, the administered dose is altered for a newly enrolled patient or cohort of patients, in accordance with the toxicity outcomes previously obtained in the trial; thus, these designs can be regarded as outcome adaptive (see, e.g., Cheung 2005, Chang 2008a, b, Chow and Chang 2011a, b, and Pong and Chow 2011) or response adaptive (see, e.g., Hu and Rosenberger 2006). In addition, dose-finding designs for MTD determination can be classified as algorithm-/rule-based or model-based designs depending on the modeling of the dose–toxicity relationship (see, e.g., Lin and Shih 2001; Edler and Burkholder 2006), or as algorithm-/rule-based, model-based, or model-assisted designs (see, e.g., Zhou et al. 2018a, b). These can also be further classified into nonparametric or parametric designs (see, e.g., Ivanova 2006; Tighiouart and Rogatko 2006). Moreover, by focusing on the dose and toxicity data utilization, a given design can be classified as a memoryless design or a design with memory (O'Quigley and Zohar 2006; Braun and Alonzo 2011).

A number of dose-finding designs for phase I/II trials primarily evaluating both toxicity and efficacy have also been developed (see, e.g., Yuan et al. 2016, in which a large number of Bayesian designs for phase I/II clinical trials are introduced with many real applications and numerical examples; O'Quigley et al. 2017, in which state-of-the-art designs for early-phase trials are provided in detail; and Hirakawa et al. 2018, in which various modern dose-finding designs for drug combinations and MTAs are discussed, along with their software implementations and some recent advanced topics).

The present manuscript is intended to constitute a brief guidebook to theory and practice that allows readers to effectively understand the core concepts and methods of dose-finding designs for early-phase cancer clinical trials. The remainder of this book is organized as follows. Chapter 2 overviews rule-based designs considering toxicity alone, including the well-known 3 + 3 design, as this design is most frequently used in practice owing to its easy implementation and transparency. Chapter 3 focuses on model-based designs, with emphasis on their standard bearer, the continual reassessment method (O'Quigley et al. 1990); this chapter is included because model-based designs usually have superior performance to rule-based designs. Chapter 4 covers model-assisted designs; these designs attract considerable attention because they possess not only the simplicity and transparency of rule-based designs but also the superior performance of model-based designs. Chapter 5 outlines designs considering both toxicity and efficacy, because the dose having the highest efficacy with admissible toxicity cannot always be determined by primarily evaluating the toxicity alone and determining the MTD, as is the case for MTAs or IAs. Finally, Chap. 6 describes several recent designs and topics related to early-phase IA trials, in which the optimal dose of an IA can be found by considering the immune response outcome in addition to the toxicity and efficacy outcomes.

References

Berry, S.M., Carlin, B.P., Lee, J.J., Müller, P.: Chapter 3. Phase I studies. In: Berry, S.M., Carlin, B.P., Lee, J.J., Müller, P. (eds.) Bayesian Adaptive Methods for Clinical Trials, First Edition, pp. 87–135. Chapman and Hall/CRC Press, Boca Raton, FL (2010)

Braun, T.M., Alonzo, T.A.: Beyond the 3+3 method: expanded algorithms for dose-escalation in phase I oncology trials of two agents. Clin. Trials **8**(3), 247–259 (2011)

Chang, M.: Adaptive Design Theory and Implementation Using SAS and R, 1st edn. Chapman and Hall/CRC Press, Boca Raton, FL (2008a)

Chang, M.: Classical and Adaptive Clinical Trial Designs Using ExpDesign Studio, 1st edn. John Wiley & Sons, Hoboken, NJ (2008b)

Cheung, Y.K.: Coherence principles in dose-finding studies. Biometrika **92**(4), 863–873 (2005)

Chevret, S.: Statistical Methods for Dose-Finding Experiments, 1st edn. John Wiley & Sons, Chichester (2006)

Chow, S.-C., Chang, M.: Adaptive Design Methods in Clinical Trials, 2nd edn. Chapman and Hall/CRC Press, Boca Raton, FL (2011a)

Chow, S.-C., Chang, M.: Chapter 5. Adaptive dose-escalation trials. In: Chow, S.-C., Chang, M. (eds.) Adaptive Design Methods in Clinical Trials, Second Edition, pp. 89–104. Chapman and Hall/CRC Press, Boca Raton, FL (2011b)

Cohen, L., de Moor, C., Amato, R.J.: The association between treatment-specific optimism and depressive symptomatology in patients enrolled in a phase I cancer clinical trial. Cancer **91**(10), 1949–1955 (2001)

Couzin-Frankel, J.: Cancer immunotherapy. Science **324**(6165), 1432–1433 (2013)

Crowley, J., Hoering, A.: Handbook of Statistics in Clinical Oncology, 3rd edn. Chapman and Hall/CRC Press, Boca Raton, FL (2012)

Daugherty, C., Ratain, M.J., Grochowski, E., Stocking, C., Kodish, E., Mick, R., Siegler, M.: Perceptions of cancer patients and their physicians involved in phase I trials. J. Clin. Oncol. **13**(5), 1062–1072 (1995)

Edler, L., Burkholder, I.: Chapter 1. Overview of phase I trials. In: Crowley, J., Ankerst, D.P. (eds.) Handbook of Statistics in Clinical Oncology, Second Edition, pp. 1–29. Chapman and Hall/CRC Press, Boca Raton, FL (2006)

Eisenhauer, E.A., O'Dwyer, P.J., Christian, M., Humphrey, J.S.: Phase I clinical trial design in cancer drug development. J. Clin. Oncol. **18**(3), 684–692 (2000)

Green, S., Benedetti, J., Crowley, J.: Clinical Trials in Oncology, 2nd edn. Chapman and Hall/CRC Press, Boca Raton, FL (2003)

Hirakawa, A., Sato, H., Daimon, T., Matsui, S.: Modern Dose-Finding Designs for Cancer Phase I Trials: Drug Combinations and Molecularly Targeted Agents. Springer, Tokyo (2018)

Horstmann, E., McCabe, M.S., Grochow, L., Yamamoto, S., Rubinstein, L., Budd, T., Shoemaker, D., Emanuel, E.J., Grady, C.: Risks and benefits of phase 1 oncology trials, 1991 through 2002. N. Engl. J. Med. **352**(9), 895–904. Correspondence: phase 1 clinical trials oncology. N. Engl. J. Med. **352**(23), 2451–2453 (2005)

Hu, F., Rosenberger, W.F.: The Theory of Response-Adaptive Randomization in Clinical Trials. John Wiley & Sons, Hoboken, NJ (2006)

Ivanova, A.: Dose-finding in oncology-nonparametric methods. In: Ting, N. (ed.) Dose Finding in Drug Development, 1st edn, pp. 49–58. Springer, New York, NY (2006)

Kurzrock, R., Benjamin, R.S.: Risks and benefits of phase 1 oncology trials, revisited. N. Engl. J. Med. **352**(9), 930–932 (2005)

Lin, Y., Shih, W.J.: Statistical properties of the traditional algorithm-based designs for phase I cancer clinical trials. Biostatistics **2**(2), 203–215 (2001)

Morrissey, K.M., Yuraszeck, T.M., Li, C.-C., Zhang, Y., Kasichayanula, S.: Immunotherapy and novel combinations in oncology: current landscape, challenges, and opportunities. Clin. Transl. Sci. **9**(2), 89–104 (2016)

O'Quigley, J., Chevret, S.: Methods for dose finding studies in cancer clinical trials: a review. Statist. Med. **10**(11), 1647–1664 (1991)

O'Quigley, J., Iasonos, A., Bornkamp, B.: Handbook of Methods for Designing, Monitoring, and Analyzing Dose-Finding Trials, 1st edn. Chapman and Hall/CRC Press, Boca Raton, FL (2017)

O'Quigley, J., Pepe, M., Fisher, L.: Continual reassessment method: a practical design for phase 1 clinical trials in cancer. Biometrics **46**(1), 33–48 (1990)

O'Quigley, J., Zohar, S.: Experimental designs for phase I and phase I/II dose-finding studies. Br. J. Cancer **94**(5), 609–613 (2006)

Paoletti, X., Baron, B., Schöffski, P., Fumoleau, P., Lacombe, D., Marreaud, S., Sylvester, R.: Using the continual reassessment method: lessons learned from an EORTC phase I dose finding study. Eur. J. Cancer **42**(10), 1362–1368 (2006)

Paoletti, X., Le Tourneau, C., Verweij, J., Siu, L.L., Seymour, L., Postel-Vinay, S., Collette, L., Rizzo, E., Ivy, P., Olmos, D., Massard, C., Lacombe, D., Kaye, S.B., Soria, J.C.: Defining dose-limiting toxicity for phase 1 trials of molecularly targeted agents: results of a DLT-TARGETT international survey. Eur. J. Cancer **50**(12), 2050–2056 (2014)

Pong, A., Chow, S.-C.: Handbook of Adaptive Designs in Pharmaceutical and Clinical Development. Chapman and Hall/CRC Press, Boca Raton, FL (2011)

Postel-Vinay, S., Aspeslagh, S., Lanoy, E., Robert, C., Soria, J.C., Marabelle, A.: Challenges of phase 1 clinical trials evaluating immune checkpoint-targeted antibodies. Ann. Oncol. **27**(2), 214–224 (2016)

Potter, D.M.: Phase I studies of chemotherapeutic agents in cancer patients: a review of the designs. J. Biopharm. Stat. **16**(5), 579–604 (2006)

Rosenberger, W.F., Haines, L.M.: Competing designs for phase I clinical trials: a review. Statist. Med. **21**(18), 2757–2770 (2002)

Storer, B.E.: Design and analysis of phase I clinical trials. Biometrics **45**(3), 925–937 (1989)

Tighiouart, M., Rogatko, A.: Dose-finding in Oncology-Parametric Methods. In: Ting, N. (ed.) Dose Finding in Drug Development, 1st edn, pp. 59–72. Springer, New York, NY (2006)

Ting, N.: Dose Finding in Drug Development. Springer, New York, NY (2006)

Tomamichel, M., Jaime, H., Degrate, A., de Jong, J., Pagani, O., Cavalli, F., Sessa, C.: Proposing phase I studies: patients', relatives', nurses' and specialists' perceptions. Ann. Oncol. **11**(3), 289–294 (2000)

Wang, C., Rosner, G.L., Roden, R.B.S.: A Bayesian design for phase I cancer therapeutic vaccine trials. Stat. Med. (2018). https://doi.org/10.1002/sim.8021

Yan, F., Thall, P.F., Lu, K.H., Gilbert, M.R., Yuan, Y.: Phase I-II clinical trial design: a state-of-the-art paradigm for dose finding. Ann. Oncol. **29**(3), 694–699 (2018)

Yin, G.: Clinical Trial Design: Bayesian and Frequentist Adaptive Methods. John Wiley & Sons, Hoboken, NJ (2012)

Yuan, Y., Nguyen, H., Thall, P.: Bayesian Designs for Phase I-II Clinical Trials. Chapman and Hall/CRC Press, Boca Raton, FL (2016)

Zhou, H., Yuan, Y., Nie, L.: Accuracy, safety, and reliability of novel phase I trial designs. Clin. Cancer. Res. (2018a). https://doi.org/10.1158/1078-0432.CCR-18-0168

Zhou, H., Murray, T.A., Pan, H., Yuan, Y.: Comparative review of novel model-assisted designs for phase I clinical trials. Statist. Med. **37**(14), 2208–2222 (2018b)

Chapter 2
Rule-Based Designs Considering Toxicity Alone

Abstract The primary objective of a phase I trial for an anticancer agent is to determine the maximum tolerated dose (MTD), which is defined as the dose having a toxicity (in particular, the dose-limiting toxicity) probability closest to the prespecified target toxicity probability level. Thus, dose-finding designs for phase I trials usually focus on the frequency or incidence of toxicity alone. Traditionally, dose-finding designs can be broadly classified as rule-/algorithm- or model-based designs. Rule-based designs identify the MTD by relying on prespecified dose escalation and de-escalation rules, whereas model-based designs estimate the MTD by fitting a model assumed to reflect the monotonic dose–toxicity relationship to the corresponding data. In this chapter, we focus on rule-based designs. In particular, we describe the $3 + 3$ design and its variations, because this is the most common rule-based design used in practice. However, we also emphasize the limitations of the $3 + 3$ design, because it poorly identifies the MTD despite its simplicity and transparency. With this in mind, we then overview alternative rule-based designs that can improve the performance of the $3 + 3$ design and discuss some related topics.

Keywords Maximum tolerated dose (MTD) · Algorithm-based designs · $3 + 3$ design

2.1 Introduction

Traditionally, the designs used to find maximum tolerated doses (MTDs) in oncological phase I clinical trials, in which toxicity is primarily evaluated, can be classified as rule- or model-based (see, e.g., Lin and Shih 2001; Edler and Burkholder 2006; Le Tourneau et al. 2009). The two design types originate from two different definitions of the MTD, which yield two different philosophies toward phase I trial design (see Rosenberger and Haines 2002; Ivanova (2006a, b). In one definition, the MTD is defined as the dose immediately below the lowest dose with an unacceptable toxicity probability level, denoted by Γ_T'. In the other definition, the MTD is defined as the dose at which the toxicity probability is equal to the maximum acceptable toxicity probability level, denoted by Γ_T. The maximum acceptable toxicity probability level

© The Author(s), under exclusive licence to Springer Japan KK 2019
T. Daimon et al., *Dose-Finding Designs for Early-Phase
Cancer Clinical Trials*, JSS Research Series in Statistics,
https://doi.org/10.1007/978-4-431-55585-8_2

is taken as lower than the unacceptable toxicity probability level; that is, $\Gamma_T < \Gamma_T'$. In the former definition, the MTD is viewed as a statistic; thus, it is observed and identified through dose escalation or de-escalation. In the latter definition, the MTD is viewed as a parameter; thus, it is estimated by fitting a model assumed to reflect the monotonic dose–toxicity relationship to the corresponding data, as well as through dose escalation or de-escalation.

Here, we focus on rule-based designs primarily considering toxicity alone that have been often used for traditional chemotherapeutic or cytotoxic agent trials. Rule-based designs originated from an up-and-down (UD) design (von Békésy 1947; Dixon and Mood 1948) according to which the agent dose is escalated if no toxicity is observed and de-escalated otherwise. The UD design concentrates the treatment distribution around the dose at which the toxicity probability is equal to 0.5 and, consequently, estimates this quantile of the underlying tolerance distribution, i.e., the median threshold. The UD design was previously used to analyze auditory thresholds or to test explosive sensitivity. Attempts were subsequently made to improve the UD design or to develop various related designs.

In this chapter, we overview the $3 + 3$ design and others, along with their dose-finding algorithms. Unless specifically noted, it is assumed that the aim of a phase I trial with a prespecified maximum sample size is MTD identification for an agent among increasing ordered doses $d_1 < \cdots < d_K$ corresponding to $1, \ldots, K$ dose levels. These dose levels are prespecified using the modified Fibonacci method or other methods in a manner that includes the true MTD (see, e.g., Collins et al. 1986; Edler and Burkholder 2006). It is also assumed that dose escalation begins from the lowest dose d_1 for safety considerations, and that the MTD is not identified from the trial if the dose escalation is stopped when the MTD is judged to be below d_1 or at/above the highest dose d_K. In either of these two cases, the protocol might include an option to add a dose level.

2.2 $3 + 3$ Designs

2.2.1 Overview

The so-called "$3 + 3$ (cohort) design" (Carter 1973; Storer 1989) is the most widely used conventional design for oncological phase I trials (see, e.g., Geller 1984; Smith et al. 1996; Rogatko et al. 2007; Le Tourneau et al. 2009; Paoletti et al. 2015). For example, according to Paoletti et al. (2015), this design has been used for MTD identification in more than 95% of published phase I trials. However, although we introduce the $3 + 3$ design here because of its conventional use in practice, we do not definitively recommend its use, as the statistical community agrees on its limitations (discussed below).

2.2.2 Dose-Finding Algorithm

Some algorithms for the 3 + 3 design have been developed (see, e.g., Korn et al. 1994; Ahn 1998; Edler and Burkholder 2006; Berry et al. 2010). The following algorithm is a version without dose de-escalation:

Step 1 Enroll a cohort of three patients, treat them at the kth dose level for $k = 1, \ldots, K$, and evaluate whether each of the three patients experiences toxicity.

(1a) If none of the three patients experience toxicity, escalate the dose to the next highest dose level ($k \to k + 1$) and go to Step 1.

(1b) If one of the three patients experiences toxicity, stay at the current dose level and go to Step 2.

(1c) If at least two patients experience toxicity, go to Step 3.

Step 2 Enroll a cohort of another three patients, treat them at the same dose level as that used in Step 1, and evaluate the toxicity in the same manner as in Step 1.

(2a) If one of the three to six ($= 3 + 3$) patients experiences toxicity, escalate the dose to the next highest dose level and go to Step 1.

(2b) If at least two patients of the three to six patients experience toxicity, go to Step 3.

Step 3 Determine that the dose level has exceeded the MTD and terminate the trial.

When Step 3 is reached, there are some possible paths toward MTD identification (see, e.g., Fig. 2.1).

The algorithm described above can be considered to be a truncated version of the group up-and-down design (GUD, see Sect. 2.3) or a special case of the $A + B$ design (see Sect. 2.6). In addition, if (1b) and (1c) under Step 1 are replaced with "(1b) If one patient experiences toxicity, remain at the current dose level and go to Step 1" and "(1c) If at least two patients experience toxicity, de-escalate the dose to the next lowest dose level and go to Step 1," respectively, and if Steps 2 and 3 are eliminated, the result is identical to that obtained from Storer's Design D (Storer 1989). Therefore, the above design can be regarded as a revised version of Storer's Design D (Reiner et al. 1999). In this regard, Storer's Design D tends to treat patients at a dose level at which the target toxicity probability level approaches 0.33 (Storer 1993). In addition, the decision to escalate or remain at the current dose can be made via the random walk method in Storer's Design D (Durham and Flournoy 1994, 1995b). (See also He et al. 2006 for discussion of MTD estimation in the 3 + 3 design.).

Figure 2.1 shows two numerical examples of the 3 + 3 design. The numbers in the body of Fig. 2.1 represent the ratio of the number of patients with a toxic response to the number of treated patients at each dose level, while the arrows indicate the dose level corresponding to the MTD identified by the 3 + 3 design. These are

(a) Without additional cohort.				
	Cohort			
Dose level (k)	1	2	3	4 MTD
1	0/3			
2		1/3	0/3	←
3			2/3	
4				

(b) With additional cohort.				
	Cohort			
Dose level (k)	1	2	3	4 MTD
1	0/3			
2			0/3	0/3 ←
3			2/3	
4				

Fig. 2.1 Numerical examples of $3 + 3$ design

examples of the requirement for MTD determination in Step 3 of the dose-finding algorithm of the $3 + 3$ design, when treating six patients. In other words, in the two numerical examples, the MTD is defined as the highest dose level at which no more than 33% of the patients experience a toxic response among at least six treated patients. Specifically, if at least two patients experience a toxic response before the number of treated patients reaches six at a given dose level, the percentage of patients experiencing toxicity at that dose level can be considered to be higher than 33%, meaning that the dose level is in excess of the MTD; in such a scenario, the dose is not escalated. In that case, the MTD is considered to be the dose level immediately below that level. If the number of patients treated at this dose level reaches six, this level is finally declared to be the MTD. If the number of patients is only three, three more patients are enrolled and treated at the dose level of interest. If the MTD definition is then satisfied, the dose level of interest is declared to be the MTD; otherwise, the search for the MTD continues at the next lowest dose level. This process is repeated until the MTD definition is satisfied at a certain dose level. However, if the MTD is observed to be exceeded by the initial dose level, the trial is stopped for safety reasons, with no dose being recommended, that is, the MTD is lower than the prespecified candidate doses.

In Fig. 2.1a, the dose was escalated according to the dose-finding algorithm of the $3 + 3$ design, for which two of the three patients had a toxic response at the third dose level. Six patients had already been treated at the dose level immediately below this level, i.e., the second dose level. Therefore, the second dose level was declared to be the MTD without enrolment of additional cohorts. Meanwhile, in Fig. 2.1b, when a toxic response was observed in two of the three patients at the third dose level, six patients had not yet been treated at the second dose level. Thus, addition of a fourth cohort was required to determine the MTD, yielding the result that the second dose level is the MTD.

2.2.3 Some Issues

The main advantages of the $3 + 3$ design are that it is safe and easy to implement (see, e.g., Le Tourneau et al. 2009), and that, through the accrual of three patients per dose level, it provides additional information on the between-patient variability of the pharmacokinetics or pharmacodynamics. However, the major disadvantages of this design, at least for cytotoxic agents, have been noted by Ratain et al. (1993) and discussed quantitatively by, e.g., Reiner et al. (1999), Lin and Shih (2001), and Ivanova (2006b). Reiner et al. (1999) highlighted the problematic aspects by noting the high probability that the 3 + 3 design algorithm terminates without correctly identifying the MTD. In other words, there is a high probability that any MTDs determined when the algorithm terminates after only a small number of subjects have been studied are incorrect. Consequently, a large proportion of patients will be treated at low, possibly subtherapeutic, dose levels below the recommended dose in the phase II trials, especially if the selected starting dose level is far below the true MTD. Similarly, based on a number of real-world clinical trial scenarios, Lin and Shih (2001) noted that the target toxicity probability level of the 3 + 3 design is lower than 33% (which is the level usually believed to be the case by clinicians) and, in actuality, is close to 0.2. Ivanova (2006b) explicitly proved that the target toxicity probability level of the 3 + 3 design is between 0.16 and 0.27, on average. Furthermore, numerous simulation results drawn from comparative analyses of the performance of a variety of designs in oncological phase I trials have indicated that, compared to other designs, the 3 + 3 design is inferior for MTD determination and for treatment of patients at doses close to the MTD (Zohar and O'Quigley 2009). Therefore, it is justifiable to assert that there are no statistical grounds for actively supporting the 3+3 design (in this regard, O'Quigley 2009's commentary of Bailey 2009 is also notable). Therefore, the 3 + 3 design should no longer be used for phase I trials (Paoletti et al. 2015).

2.2.4 Software for Implementation

We can calculate all possible trial pathways for the 3 + 3 design, together with their occurrence probability, using the `threep3` function of the `bcrm` R package. If the candidate doses, their true toxicity probabilities, and the starting dose level are supplied, this function allows confirmation of the operating characteristics without simulation. For example, the experimentation probability at each dose level, the probability of each dose level being identified as the MTD, the average number of patients dosed at each level, and the average number of toxicities experienced at each dose level can be confirmed. It should be noted that the 3 + 3 design here incorporates the following dose escalation and de-escalation rules to the next dose level for subsequent cohorts:

- If none of the three patients or at most one of the six patients in the current cohort experience toxicity and the next highest dose level has not yet been tested, escalate the dose to the next highest dose level.
- If one of the three patients experiences toxicity at the current dose level, remain at this dose level.

- If at least two of the three to six patients experience toxicity at the current dose level and fewer than six patients have been treated at the next lowest level, de-escalate the dose to the next lowest dose level.
- If none of the above rules are satisfied, the trial is terminated. If the current dose level yields, at most, one patient experiencing toxicity, this is claimed to be the MTD; otherwise, the dose level below is deemed to be the MTD.
- If the dose is escalated outside the prespecified candidate doses, the MTD is determined to be the largest dose.

```
# Candidate doses
dose <- c(1,2.5,5,10)

# True probabilities of toxicity
p.tox0 <- c(0.100,0.170,0.333,0.400)

# Implementation
design.threep3 <- threep3(truep=p.tox0,start=1,dose=dose)
print(design.threep3)

                    Mean Minimum Maximum
Sample size 13.68408        3      24

                            Doses
                      < 1      1      2      3       4
Experimentation proportion   NA  0.374  0.332  0.22  0.0740
Recommendation proportion  0.0991 0.226 0.412  0.17  0.0928

                       Probability of DLT
                      [0,0.2] (0.2,0.4] (0.4,0.6]
Experimentation proportion   0.706      0.294        0
Recommendation proportion*   0.638      0.263        0
                       Probability of DLT
                      (0.6,0.8] (0.8,1]
Experimentation proportion       0       0
Recommendation proportion*       0       0

* Among those trials that recommend an MTD

                            Doses
                        1      2      3      4
Average number of patients 4.290  4.640  3.46  1.290
Average number of DLTs      0.429  0.789  1.15  0.516
```

2.3 Group Up-and-Down Design

2.3.1 Overview

The GUD design constitutes the basis of rule-based designs. Anderson et al. (1946) first proposed the GUD design (Gezmu and Flournoy 2006); this research was extended by, e.g., Wetherill (1963), Tsutakawa (1967a, b), and Durham et al. (1997).

Further development was performed by other researchers, e.g., Ivanova et al. (2003), Ivanova et al. (2006b), and Gezmu and Flournoy (2006).

2.3.2 Dose-Finding Algorithm

The concept behind the GUD design is to treat patients at and around the dose at which the toxicity probability is equal to a prespecified target toxicity probability level. Let Y_T denote the binary random variable for the toxicity outcome, where $Y_T = 1$ and 0 indicate toxicity and the absence of toxicity, respectively; X is the random variable for the dose that satisfies $X \in \{d_1, \ldots, d_K\}$; C_{GUD} is the cohort size; $C^{\downarrow}$ and $C^{\uparrow}$ are two integers such that $0 \leq C^{\downarrow} < C^{\uparrow} < C_{GUD}$; and $n_T(d_k)$ is the number of patients experiencing toxicity in the cohort of patients treated at dose level k. Thus, $n_T(d_k)$ is a random variable assumed to have a binomial distribution with parameters C_{GUD} and $Pr(Y_T = 1 | X = d_k)$, denoted by $Bin(C_{GUD}, Pr(Y_T = 1 | X = d_k))$.

The dose-finding algorithm of the GUD design is as follows:

Step 1 Enroll a cohort of C_{GUD} patients, treat them at the kth dose level for $k = 1, \ldots, K$, and evaluate whether each of the C_{GUD} patients experiences toxicity.

(1a) If $n_T(d_k) \leq C^{\downarrow}$, escalate the dose to the next highest dose level ($k \to k + 1$) and repeat Step 1.

(1b) If $C^{\downarrow} < n_T(d_k) < C^{\uparrow}$, remain at the current dose level and repeat Step 1.

(1c) If $n_T(d_k) \geq C^{\uparrow}$, de-escalate the dose to the next lowest dose level and repeat Step 1.

To facilitate easy understanding of the various designs mentioned below, we refer to the GUD design, denoting this algorithm as $GUD(C_{GUD}, C^{\downarrow}, C^{\uparrow})$.

2.3.3 Some Issues

The MTD can be estimated using a statistical procedure, e.g., isotonic regression (see, e.g., Stylianou and Flournoy 2002; Gezmu and Flournoy 2006). To find the MTD, values of C, $C^{\downarrow}$, and $C^{\uparrow}$ must be chosen. Letting Γ_T denote the prespecified target toxicity probability level, these values are chosen such that Γ_T approximately satisfies the following equation:

$$Pr\left\{Bin(C_{GUD}, \Gamma_T) \leq C^{\downarrow}\right\} = Pr\left\{Bin(C_{GUD}, \Gamma_T) \geq C^{\uparrow}\right\}. \qquad (2.1)$$

Values of C_{GUD}, $C^{\downarrow}$, and $C^{\uparrow}$ are provided for a given value of Γ_T by Gezmu and Flournoy (2006). It should be noted that the GUD design is based on information on the toxicity outcome obtained from the current cohort of patients only.

The so-called "escalation design" can be regarded as a special case of the GUD design. The escalation design can be obtained by replacing C_{GUD}, $C^{\downarrow}$, and $C^{\uparrow}$ in the GUD design with C_E, $C^{\uparrow\uparrow}$, and $C^{\uparrow\uparrow} + 1$, respectively, i.e., to obtain $GUD(C_E, C^{\uparrow\uparrow}, C^{\uparrow\uparrow} + 1)$, where C_E is the cohort size and $C^{\uparrow\uparrow}$ is a prespecified integer. The dose-finding algorithm terminates when it calls for dose de-escalation, and the MTD is identified as the dose level below that with $n_T(d_k) > C^{\uparrow\uparrow}$.

2.4 Two-Stage Designs

2.4.1 Overview

Storer (1989) proposed two two-stage designs by combining variations of up-and-down designs presented by Wetherill (1963) and Wetherill and Levitt (1965). Here, we describe the more commonly used of these two two-stage designs, referred to as "Design BD" by Storer (1989).

2.4.2 Dose-Finding Algorithm

The Design BD dose-finding algorithm is as follows:

Step 1 Enroll one patient, treat him/her at the kth dose level for $k = 1, \ldots, K$, and evaluate whether he/she experiences toxicity.

   (1a) If no patient has had experienced toxicity, escalate the dose to the next highest dose level ($k \rightarrow k + 1$) and repeat Step 1.
   (1b) If all patients have had experienced toxicity, de-escalate the dose to the next lowest dose level and repeat Step 1.
   (1c) If at least one patient has had experienced toxicity and at least one patient has not had experienced toxicity, and if the current patient has not had experienced toxicity, go to Step 2; otherwise, de-escalate the dose to the next lowest dose level ($k \rightarrow k - 1$) and go to Step 2.

Step 2 Enroll a cohort of another three patients, treat them at the same dose level as that of Step 1, and evaluate whether each of the three patients experiences toxicity.

   (2a) If none of the three patients experience toxicity, escalate the dose to the next highest dose level and repeat Step 2.
   (2b) If one of the three patients experiences toxicity, remain at the current dose level and repeat Step 2.
   (2c) If at least two patients experience toxicity, de-escalate the dose to the next lowest dose level and repeat Step 2.

At the end of Step 2 (the second stage), a logistic model is fit to the data and the MTD is estimated using the maximum likelihood or Bayesian method. Note that procedures for interval estimation of the MTD were constructed by Storer (1993).

2.4.3 Some Issues

Step 1 (the first stage) satisfies the requirement for heterogeneity in the toxicity outcome. Step 2 (the second stage) is partially similar to the $3 + 3$ design and targets a toxicity probability level of $1/3$. This step can be regarded as a discretized version of a stochastic approximation design as described by Robbins and Monro (1951), with spaced dose levels.

2.5 Accelerated Titration Designs

2.5.1 Overview

A family of accelerated titration (AT) designs was proposed by Simon et al. (1997). The main features that distinguish these designs from others are that the AT designs allow clinical investigators

1. to include a rapid initial escalation stage, called an accelerated stage, where one patient is treated per dose level;
2. to account for not only dose-limiting and unacceptable toxicity, but also moderate toxicity;
3. to have options for intrapatient dose modification; and
4. to analyze trial results using a model with intra- and interpatient variation parameters in the toxicity and cumulative toxicity.

2.5.2 Dose-Finding Algorithm

The family of AT designs is implemented as follows:

Design 1 is the $3 + 3$ design (see Sect. 2.2).
Design 2 continues the accelerated phase unless one patient experiences dose-limiting toxicity (DLT) or two patients experience moderate toxicity during their first course of treatment. If so, the escalation phase switches to Design 1 with 40% dose-step increments.

Design 3 employs the same dose-finding algorithm as Design 2, but with double dose steps (100% dose-step increments) in the accelerated phase.

Design 4 has the same dose-finding algorithm as Design 3, but continues the accelerated phase unless one patient experiences DLT or two patients experience moderate toxicity in "any" course of treatment.

2.5.3 Some Issues

To achieve feature 1 listed in the overview (Sect. 2.5.1), a single patient cohort per dose level is used for the accelerated stage in the AT designs (except for Design 1). Such a single-cohort stage allows trial acceleration and reduction of the number of patients to whom low doses are allocated. To achieve feature 2, the AT designs utilize the toxicity grade evaluated using the National Cancer Institute Common Terminology Criteria for Adverse Events (NCI-CTCAE, see Sect. 1.2.1), for dose finding. Specifically, these designs use the first onset of first-course DLT to trigger the switch, as in the two-stage design proposed by Storer (1989) (see Sect. 2.4) and utilize the first-course moderate toxicity to provide an added element of caution. In particular, these designs use the second onset of moderate toxicity in a heterogeneous population in a phase I trial to determine whether any moderate toxicity is related to the agent. For feature 3, to provide the opportunity for each patient to be treated at the potentially active dose, Designs 2–4 can personalize the dose for any patient remaining on the trial. Two options (A and B) are given by Simon et al.(1997). In option A, there is no intrapatient dose escalation. If a patient experiences moderate toxicity, the same dose level is maintained; however, if a patient experiences dose-limiting or more severe toxicity and remains on the study, the dose is de-escalated. In option B, if a patient experiences none–mild toxicity at the current dose level during the current course, the dose is escalated for the next course; otherwise, the procedure in option A is adopted. To realize feature 4, the model used in the AT designs is a generalization of the K_{max} model (Sheiner et al., 1989; Sheiner et al. 1991) or the model presented by Chou and Talalay (1984).

2.5.4 Software for Implementation

Readers can employ the AT designs using a Microsoft Excel macro for dose allocation and the S-PLUS program for analysis of these designs, available at https://linus.nci.nih.gov/~brb/Methodologic.htm.

2.6   *A* + *B* **Design**

2.6.1   *Overview*

Lin and Shih (2001) proposed the $A + B$ design based on investigation of some key statistical properties. This design has the advantages that the required number of patients is allocated by stopping the dose escalation, similar to the escalation design; and that resources are conserved at lower doses through allocation of more patients at or close to the MTD, similar to the GUD design. As mentioned by Ivanova (2006b), the $A + B$ design can also be regarded as the GUD design with a cohort of size A, i.e., $\mathrm{GUD}(A, C^{\downarrow}, C^{\uparrow})$, that nests the escalation design with a cohort of size $A + B$, i.e., $\mathrm{GUD}(A + B, C^{\uparrow\uparrow}, C^{\uparrow\uparrow} + 1)$, where $C^{\downarrow}$, $C^{\uparrow}$, and $C^{\uparrow\uparrow}$ are integers such that $0 \leq C^{\downarrow} < C^{\uparrow} \leq A$, $C^{\uparrow} - C^{\downarrow} \geq 2$, and $C^{\downarrow} \leq C^{\uparrow\uparrow} < A + B$. Whenever the former design requires that the current dose be maintained, the process switches to the latter design.

2.6.2   *Dose-Finding Algorithm*

Let $n_{\mathrm{T},A}(d_k)$ and $n_{\mathrm{T},A+B}(d_k)$ denote the number of patients experiencing toxicity in cohorts of sizes A and $A + B$ (when B additional patients are added to the cohort), respectively.

The dose-finding algorithm of the $A + B$ design without dose de-escalation is as follows:

Step 1   Enroll a cohort of A patients, treat them at the kth dose level for $k = 1, \ldots, K$, and evaluate whether each of the A patients experiences toxicity.

    (1a)   If $n_{\mathrm{T},A}(d_k) \leq C^{\downarrow}$, escalate the dose to the next highest level and repeat Step 1.

    (1b)   If $C^{\downarrow} < n_{\mathrm{T},A}(d_k) < C^{\uparrow}$, remain at the current dose level and go to Step 2.

    (1c)   If $n_{\mathrm{T},A}(d_k) \geq C^{\uparrow}$, go to Step 3.

Step 2   Enroll a cohort of another B patients, treat them at the same dose level as in Step 1, and evaluate the toxicity in the same manner as in Step 1.

    (2a)   If $n_{\mathrm{T},A+B}(d_k) \leq C^{\uparrow\uparrow}$, escalate the dose to the next highest dose level and go to Step 1.

    (2b)   If $n_{\mathrm{T},A+B}(d_k) > C^{\uparrow\uparrow}$, go to Step 3.

Step 3   Determine that the dose level has exceeded the MTD and terminate the trial.

If Step 3 is reached, the dose level below that where $n_{\mathrm{T},A}(d_k) \geq C^{\uparrow}$ or $n_{\mathrm{T},A+B}(d_k) > C^{\uparrow\uparrow}$ is identified as the MTD.

2.6.3 Some Issues

The $3 + 3$ design (see Sect. 2.2) is a special version of the $A + B$ design. In fact, the $3 + 3$ design can be expressed as a combination of $\text{GUD}(A = 3, C^{\downarrow} = 0, C^{\uparrow} = 2)$ and $\text{GUD}(A + B = 6, C^{\downarrow} = 1, C^{\uparrow} + 1 = 2)$.

Note that Ivanova (2006b) has discussed the GUD, escalation, and $A + B$ designs in terms of their operating characteristics and provided recommendations for setting of their design parameters.

2.6.4 Software for Implementation

Wheeler et al. (2016) developed a web application for investigating the operating characteristics of the $A + B$ design. This application is available using the Shiny package. Readers can access the application at https://graham-wheeler.shinyapps. io/AplusB/ and download the R code from GitHub at https://github.com/graham-wheeler/AplusB.

When the candidate doses, their true toxicity probabilities, the cohort sizes, thresholds for dose escalation and de-escalation, and an indicator of whether dose de-escalation is permitted are provided, this application facilitates confirmation of the design- and scenario-specific operating characteristics. In addition, the trial operating characteristics, such as the sample size distribution, probability of experimentation at each dose level, probability of recommending each dose level as the MTD, and DLT rate distribution, can be plotted. For example, we can obtain the plots shown in Fig. 2.2 using this application.

2.7 Best-of-5 Design

2.7.1 Overview

The best-of-5 design (Storer 2001) can be regarded as a combination of $\text{GUD}(3, 0, 3)$, $\text{GUD}(4, 1, 3)$, and $\text{GUD}(5, 2, 3)$.

2.7.2 Dose-Finding Algorithm

Let $n_{T,3}(d_k)$ and $n_{T,3+1}(d_k)$ denote the number of patients experiencing toxicity in cohorts of sizes 3 and $3 + 1$ ($=$ total 4, when one more patient is added to the cohort), respectively, and $n_{T,3+1+1}(d_k)$ denote the number of patients experiencing toxicity

Plot of trial operating characteristics

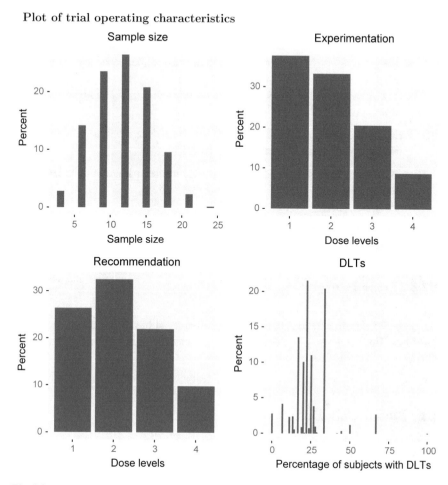

Fig. 2.2 Plots of operating characteristics of $A + B$ design

in a cohort of size $3 + 1 + 1$ ($= 4 + 1 =$ total 5, when one more patient is added to the cohort of size 4).

The dose-finding algorithm of the best-of-5 design is as follows:

Step 1 Enroll a cohort of three patients, treat them at the kth dose level for $k = 1, \ldots, K$, and evaluate whether each of the three patients experiences toxicity.

(1a) If $n_{T,3}(d_k) \leq 0$, escalate the dose to the next highest dose level and repeat Step 1.

(1b) If $0 < n_{T,3}(d_k) < 3$, remain at the current dose level and go to Step 2.

(1c) If $n_{T,3}(d_k) \geq 3$, go to Step 4.

Step 2 Enroll and treat one more patient at the same dose level as in Step 1, and evaluate whether he/she experiences toxicity.

(2a) If $n_{T,3+1}(d_k) \leq 1$, escalate the dose to the next highest dose level and repeat Step 1.

(2b) If $1 < n_{T,3+1}(d_k) < 3$, remain at the current dose level and go to Step 3.

(2c) If $n_{T,3+1}(d_k) \geq 3$, go to Step 4.

Step 3 Enroll and treat one more patient at the same dose level as in Step 2, and evaluate whether he/she experiences toxicity.

(3a) If $n_{T,3+1+1}(d_k) \leq 2$, escalate the dose to the next highest dose level and repeat Step 1.

(3b) If $n_{T,3+1+1}(d_k) \geq 3$, go to Step 4.

Step 4 Determine that the dose level has exceeded the MTD and terminate the trial.

2.7.3 Some Issues

The best-of-5 design can be expected to treat literally at best five patients at a given dose level. This design employs relatively few patients, targeting $\Gamma_T \approx 0.4$ (see Storer 2001).

2.8 Biased-Coin Design

2.8.1 Overview

One approach to targeting any toxicity probability level is to organize patients into a group or cohort and to treat them at the corresponding dose level, as in the GUD design. Another approach is to leave the dose for the next patient unchanged if it is associated with a certain target toxicity probability level, or to escalate or de-escalate the dose otherwise, depending solely on the toxicity outcome for the current patient. Durham and Flournoy (1995a, b) proposed the biased-coin (BC) design (see also, e.g., Derman 1957; Durham and Flournoy 1994; Giovagnoli and Pintacuda 1998; Stylianou et al. 2003). In this case, it is assumed that $\Gamma_T \leq 0.5$. Otherwise, Γ_T is replaced with $1 - \Gamma_T$.

2.8.2 Dose-Finding Algorithm

The dose-finding algorithm of the BC design is as follows:

Step 1 Enroll the first patient, treat him/her at a dose level of $1, \ldots, K$, and evaluate whether he/she experiences toxicity. Enroll the subsequent patient j ($j = 2, \ldots$), treat him/her at the kth dose level, and evaluate the toxicity outcomes for him/her.

   (1a) If patient $j - 1$ experiences no toxicity, we flip a biased coin with the probability of obtaining the head side being equal to $\Gamma_T/(1 - \Gamma_T)$ and go to the appropriate following sub-step:

   (i) If the head side is obtained, escalate the dose to the next highest dose level, replace patient $j - 1$ with patient j, and go to Step 1.

   (ii) If the tail side is obtained, remain at the current dose level, replace patient $j - 1$ with j, and go to Step 1.

   (1b) If patient $j - 1$ experiences toxicity, de-escalate the dose to the next lowest dose level and repeat Step 1.

The MTD can be nonparametrically estimated as the treatment distribution mode (see, e.g., Durham and Flournoy 1995b and Giovagnoli and Pintacuda 1998), but can be also estimated through isotonic regression (see, e.g., Stylianou and Flournoy 2002), where the estimates can be obtained using the pool-adjacent-violators algorithm (see Robertson et al. 1988).

2.8.3 Some Issues

The BC design requires complete follow-up for every patient, like other designs. Thus, situations where the patient follow-up times are long compared with the interarrival times may yield long trials with delayed or refused patient entry. The accelerated biased-coin up-and-down (ABCUD) design developed by Stylianou and Follmann (2004) is one approach that does not require such a complete follow-up for the current patient. This design is equivalent to the BC design when follow-up is completed for every patient. However, when follow-up is not completed for the current patient and a newly enrolled patient is ready for enrollment, the ABCUD design treats the new patient at a dose level determined based on the outcome for the patient for whom the follow-up has most recently been completed. One problem with the ABCUD design is that partial information collected from patients for whom follow-up has not been completed is ignored. To solve to this problem, a time-to-event version of the BC design, referred to as the adaptive accelerated BC design, has recently been proposed by Jia and Braun (2011).

2.9 Cumulative Cohort Design

2.9.1 Overview

Ivanova et al. (2007) proposed a generalization of the GUD design, called the cumulative cohort (CC) design, in which the dose is unchanged if the toxicity rate at the current dose is close to Γ_T within some range δ (> 0) of the target.

2.9.2 Dose-Finding Algorithm

Let Y_T denote the binary random variable for the toxicity outcome, where $Y_T = 1$ indicates toxicity and $Y_T = 0$ otherwise. Furthermore, C_{CC} is the cohort size and $\check{\Pr}(Y_T|d_k)$ is the isotonic regression estimate (see Robertson et al. 1988) of the toxicity probability at the kth dose level. The dose-finding algorithm of the CC design is as follows:

Step 1 Enroll a cohort of C_{CC} patients, treat them at the kth dose level for $k = 1, \ldots, K$, and evaluate whether each of the C_{CC} patients experiences toxicity.

    (1a) If $\check{\Pr}(Y_T|d_k) \leq \Gamma_T - \delta$, escalate the dose to the next highest dose level and repeat Step 1.

    (1b) If $\Gamma_T - \delta < \check{\Pr}(Y_T|d_k) < \Gamma_T + \delta$, stay at the current dose level and repeat Step 1.

    (1c) If $\check{\Pr}(Y_T|d_k) \geq \Gamma_T + \delta$, de-escalate the dose to the next lowest dose level and repeat Step 1.

2.9.3 Some Issues

To maximize the number of patients to which the MTD is allocated in a trial with a moderate sample size, it is important to choose an appropriate δ. Ivanova et al. (2007) recommend use of $\delta = 0.09$ if $\Gamma_T = 0.10, 0.15, 0.20$, or 0.25; $\delta = 0.10$ if $\Gamma_T = 0.30$ or 0.35; $\delta = 0.12$ if $\Gamma_T = 0.40$; and $\delta = 0.13$ if $\Gamma_T = 0.45$ or 0.50. Another natural choice for the δ range in the CC design is δ close to 0. For example, with $\delta = 0.01$ for moderate sample sizes, the dose is repeated if the estimated toxicity rate is almost equal to Γ_T and changed otherwise.

2.9.4 Software for Implementation

Readers can use the U-design commercial online software available at https://udesign.laiyaconsulting.com/ to implement a modified version of the CC design with the following safety rules:

1. If the lowest dose level has a high chance of being above the MTD, and if at least two patients have experienced toxicity at the lowest dose in the meantime, the trial is terminated before the maximum sample size is reached.
2. If any dose level has a high chance of exceeding the MTD, and if at least two patients have experienced toxicity at dose level k for $k = 1, \ldots, K$ in the meantime, dose level k and all doses higher than k are excluded from the trial.

Using the U-design software, six mainstream designs can be compared via simulation: rule-based designs such as the $3 + 3$ design and the modified CC design, model-based designs (see Chap. 3) such as the continual reassessment method (CRM) and the Bayesian logistic regression method (BLRM), and model-assisted designs (see Chap. 4) such as the modified toxicity probability interval (mTPI) design and the mTPI-2 design.

For the modified CC design, we input the following settings: the under-dosing interval, denoted by $(0, \Gamma_T - \delta_1)$; the over-dosing interval, denoted by $(\Gamma_T + \delta_2, 1)$; and the proper-dosing interval, denoted by $[\Gamma_T - \delta_1, \Gamma_T + \delta_2]$. Here, δ_1 and δ_2 are small prespecified values, say 0.05, instead of the $\Gamma_T - \delta$, $(\Gamma_T - \delta, \Gamma_T + \delta)$, and $\Gamma_T + \delta$ thresholds for the original CC design, respectively, like the mTPI design. We also input the starting dose level, the number of dose levels, the cohort size, the maximum sample size, and the number of simulated trials.

Hence, we can obtain simulation results such as the proportion of recommendations of each dose level or no dose level as the MTD, the proportion of selected dose levels above the true MTD, and the proportion of patients experiencing toxicity, as shown in Fig. 2.3.

2.10 Pharmacologically Guided Dose Escalation Design

2.10.1 Overview

Phase I trials using some of the above designs may have long completion times, especially when the starting dose is far below the MTD and the dose increment is moderate. Acceleration of the dose escalation in phase I trials is desirable; however, this is accompanied by the risk of exposing a patient to a high dose, which may be toxic. If the treatment in question is in the form of an agent, one approach to solving the problem of safely accelerating the dose escalation is to utilize the relationships between the pharmacokinetics and pharmacodynamics (toxicodynamics), rather than the dose–toxicity relationship. Based on this concept, Collins et al. (1986) proposed

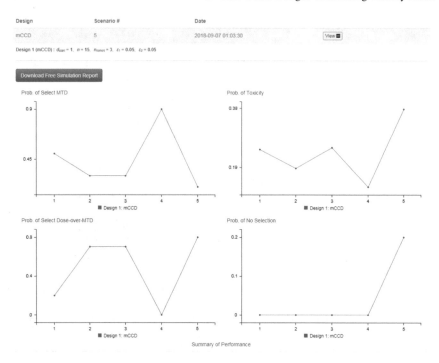

Fig. 2.3 Simulation results for CC design

the pharmacologically guided dose escalation (PGDE) design. This design focuses on the area under the curve (AUC) of the agent concentration in plasma measured over the agent exposure time, which represents the plasma cumulative exposure of the agent and is taken as a pharmacokinetic index. The toxicity is taken as the pharmacodynamic response of interest. This design assumes that toxicity can be some function of the AUC and that this relationship in animal models can be extrapolated to humans.

2.10.2 Dose-Finding Algorithm

The dose-finding algorithm of the PGDE is as follows:

Step 1 Determine the lethal dose 10% (LD_{10}) and the associated AUC in mice.

Step 2 Enroll a cohort of patients, treat them at a certain dose (e.g., the 1/10 mouse equivalent LD_{10} ($MELD_{10}$) for the first cohort), measure the AUCs, and evaluate whether each of these patients experiences toxicity.

(2a) If the average AUC for these patients does not reach some prespecified target AUC in humans that is associated with $MELD_{10}$, escalate the dose according to the distance to the target AUC and repeat Step 2.

(2b) If the average AUC for these patients reaches the target AUC or if toxicity occurs, go to Step 3.

Step 3 Terminate the trial.

2.10.3 Some Issues

There exist *advantages* and *disadvantages* of the PGDE design, including practical difficulties in observing real-time pharmacokinetic data, extrapolating preclinical data to human data, and handling interpatient pharmacokinetic variation (for details, see EORTC Pharmacokinetics and Metabolism Group 1987; Collins et al. 1990; Newell 1994).

2.11 An Overview of Other Designs and Related Topics

2.11.1 Designs for Pediatric Phase I Trials

Skolnik et al. (2008) introduced the "rolling-six" design to shorten the duration of pediatric phase I trials while avoiding the risk of toxicity (see also Hartford et al 2008; O'Quigley 2009). This design can be implemented using the aforementioned U-design software.

2.11.2 Stochastic Approximation Designs

Robbins and Monro (1951) proposed the formal stochastic approximation procedure to find the root of a regression function. The Robbins–Monro stochastic approximation was subsequently studied by, e.g., Wetherill (1963), Anbar (1984), and Wu (1985). Cheung and Elkind (2010) proposed generation of a stochastic approximation recursion based on virtual observations for dose finding. Furthermore, Cheung (2010) published a review in which he discussed the relevance of stochastic approximation to dose-finding trials.

2.11.3 Isotonic Designs

A nonparametric approach toward fully exploiting the monotonicity assumption that toxicity is increased with dose involves application of isotonic regression to all obtained data on the administered dose and toxicity outcome. Some designs using isotonic regression have been developed, for one-agent trials (see Leung and Wang 2001; Stylianou and Flournoy 2002), agent combinations (see Conaway et al. 2004; Ivanova and Wang 2006), and ordered groups (Yuan and Chappell 2004; Ivanova and Wang 2006). Furthermore, Ivanova and Flournoy (2009) previously compared several rule-based designs based on isotonic regression estimators proposed by Leung and Wang (2001), Conaway et al. (2004), and Ivanova et al. (2007).

2.11.4 Stepwise Designs

Cheung (2007) studied a class of stepwise procedures to find the MTD of a given agent, adopting a multiple test framework in which stepdown and stepup tests were used in the escalation and de-escalation stages, respectively. This approach facilitated sequential dose assignments for ethical purposes.

2.11.5 Designs for Intrapatient Multiple Doses

Fan and Wang (2007) proposed designs involving multiple doses per patient for phase I trials, and then explored their implementation as a means of improving design efficiency. They evaluated the efficiency gain acquired by changing from a single dose per patient to multiple doses per patient.

2.11.6 Designs for Ordinal Toxicity Outcome

Gordon and Willson (1992) proposed a design involving three patient accrual stages, in which one, three, or six patients are evaluated at each dose level in stage 1, 2, or 3, and the dose escalation scheme in each stage depends on toxicity grades 0–5. In addition, Paul et al. (2004) developed a multidimensional extension of Stylianou and Flournoy's estimator (Stylianou and Flournoy 2002), called the "nonparametric multidimensional isotonic regression estimator." They also developed a modified version, called the "multidimensional isotonic regression-based estimator," for estimation of a set of target quantiles from an ordinal toxicity scale, and explored a generalization of the random walk design (Durham et al. 1997) for the ordinal toxicity outcome. Paul et al. (2004) then compared their proposed estimator with the standard parametric maximum likelihood estimator obtained from a proportional odds model, in conjunction with three designs considering ordinal toxicity: that proposed by Simon et al. (1997), where Design 2 is used (see Sect. 2.5); a modified version of the three-stage design proposed by Gordon and Willson (1992); and their own proposed multistage random walk design (Paul et al. 2004). To determine whether designs considering the ordinal toxicity outcome really improve upon nonparametric designs featuring binary toxicity outcomes, Paul et al. (2004) also compared the former to the isotonic regression design proposed by Leung and Wang (2002), in which the toxicity outcomes are dichotomized for design purposes but ordinality is preserved for estimation purposes. Hence, they showed that the proposed multidimensional isotonic regression-based estimator is superior to the alternatives with regard to both accuracy and efficiency. Note that the design developed by Simon et al. (1997) was found to provide particularly efficient estimators compared to the random walk design, but had the largest number of DLTs.

2.11.7 Designs for Drug Combinations

There exist several rule-based designs to determine the maximum tolerated combination of two agents, such as the abovementioned isotonic designs and the $A + B + C$ designs (see Braun and Alonzo 2011).

References

Ahn, C.: An evaluation of phase I cancer clinical trial designs. Stat. Med. **17**(14), 1537–1549 (1998)

Anbar, D.: Stochastic approximation methods and their use in bioassay and phase I clinical trials. Commun. Stat. Theory Methods **13**(19), 2451–2467 (1984)

Anderson, T., McCarthy, P., Tukey, J.: Staircase method of sensitivity testing. Naval Ordinance Report, Statistical Research Group, Princeton University, Princeton, NJ, pp. 46–65 (1946)

Bailey, R.A.: Designs for dose-escalation trials with quantitative responses. Stat. Med. **28**(30), 3721–3738 (2009)

Berry, S.M., Carlin, B.P., Lee, J.J., Müller, P.: Chapter 3. Phase I studies. In: Berry, S.M., Carlin, B.P., Lee, J.J., Müller, P. (eds.) Bayesian Adaptive Methods for Clinical Trials, 1st edn, pp. 87–135. Chapman and Hall/CRC Press, Boca Raton, FL (2010)

Braun, T.M., Alonzo, T.A.: Beyond the 3 + 3 method: expanded algorithms for dose-escalation in phase I oncology trials of two agents. Clin. Trials **8**(3), 247–259 (2011)

Carter, S.K.: Study design principles for the clinical evaluation of new drugs as developed by the chemotherapy programme of the National Cancer Institute. In: Staquet, M.J. (ed.) The Design of Clinical Trials in Cancer Therapy, 1st edn, pp. 242–289. Editions Scientifique Europe, Brussels. (1973)

Cheung, Y.K.: Sequential implementation of stepwise procedures for identifying the maximum tolerated dose. J. Am. Stat. Assoc. **102**, 1448–1461 (2007)

Cheung, Y.K.: Stochastic approximation and modern model-based designs for dose-finding clinical trials. Stat. Sci. **25**(2), 191–201 (2010)

Cheung, Y.K., Elkind, M.S.V.: Stochastic approximation with virtual observations for dose-finding on discrete levels. Biometrika **97**(1), 109–121 (2010)

Chou, T.C., Talalay, P.: Quantitative analysis of dose-effect relationships: the combined effects of multiple drugs or enzyme inhibitors. Adv. Enzyme. Regul. **22(C)**, 27–55 (1984)

Collins, J.M., Grieshaber, C.K., Chabner, B.A.: Pharmacologically guided phase I clinical trials based upon preclinical drug development. J. Nat. Cancer Inst. **82**(16), 1321–1326 (1990)

Collins, J.M., Zaharko, D.S., Dedrick, R.L., Chabner, B.A.: Potential roles for preclinical pharmacology in phase I clinical trials. Cancer. Treat. Rep. **70**(1), 73–80 (1986)

Conaway, M.R., Dunbar, S., Peddada, S.D.: Designs for single- or multiple-agent phase I trials. Biometrics **60**(3), 661–669 (2004)

Derman, C.: Nonparametric up and down experimentation. Ann. Math. Stat. **28**(3), 795–798 (1957)

Dixon, W.J., Mood, A.M.: A method for obtaining and analyzing sensitivity data. J. Am. Stat. Assoc. **43**(241), 109–126 (1948)

Durham, S.D., Flournoy, N.: Random walks for quantile estimation. In: Gupta, S.S., Berger, J.O. (eds.) Statistical Decision Theory and Related Topics V, 1st edn, pp. 467–476. Springer, New York, NY (1994)

Durham, S.D., Flournoy, N.: Up-and-down designs I. Stationary treatment distributions. In Flournoy, N., Rosenberger, W.F. (eds.) Adaptive Designs: Papers from the Joint AMS-IMS-SIAM Summer Conference held at Mt. Holyoke College, South Hadley, MA, July 1992. IMS Lecture Notes Monograph Series, 1st edn, vol. 25, pp. 139–157. Institute of Mathematical Statistics, Hayward, CA (1995a)

Durham, S.D., Flournoy, N.: Up-and-down designs II. Exact treatment moments. In Flournoy, N., Rosenberger, W.F. (eds.) Adaptive Designs: Papers from the Joint AMS-IMS-SIAM Summer Conference held at Mt. Holyoke College, South Hadley, MA, July 1992. IMS Lecture Notes Monograph Series, 1st edn, vol. 25, pp. 158–178. Institute of Mathematical Statistics, Hayward, CA (1995b)

Durham, S.D., Flournoy, N., Rosenberger, W.F.: A random walk rule for phase I clinical trials. Biometrics **53**(2), 745–760 (1997)

Edler, L., Burkholder, I.: Chapter 1. Overview of phase I trials. In: Crowley, J., Ankerst, D.P. (eds.) Handbook of Statistics in Clinical Oncology, 2nd edn, pp. 1–29. Chapman and Hall/CRC Press, Boca Raton, FL (2006)

EORTC Pharmacokinetics and Metabolism Group: Pharmacologically guided dose escalation in phase I clinical trials: commentary and proposed guidelines. Eur. J. Cancer. Clin. Oncol. **23**(7), 1083–1087 (1987)

Fan, S.K., Wang, Y.-G.: Designs for phase I clinical trials with multiple courses of subjects at different doses. Biometrics **63**(3), 856–864 (2007)

Geller, N.L.: Design of phase I and II clinical trials in cancer: a statistician's view. Cancer Invest. **2**(6), 483–491 (1984)

Gezmu, M., Flournoy, N.: Group up-and-down designs for dose-finding. J. Stat. Plan. Inference **136**(6), 1749–1764 (2006)

Giovagnoli, A., Pintacuda, N.: Properties of frequency distributions induced by general 'up-and-down' methods for estimating quantiles. J. Stat. Plan. Inference **74**(1), 51–63 (1998)

Gordon, N.H., Willson, J.K.V.: Using toxicity grades in the design and analysis of cancer phase I clinical trials. Stat. Med. **11**(16), 2063–2075 (1992)

Hartford, C., Volchenboum, S.L., Cohn, S.L.: $3 + 3 \neq$ (Rolling) 6. J. Clin. Oncol. **26**(2), 170–171 (2008)

He, W., Liu, J., Binkowitz, B., Quan, H.: A model-based approach in the estimation of the maximum tolerated dose in phase I cancer clinical trials. Stat. Med. **25**(12), 2027–2042 (2006)

Ivanova, A.: Dose-finding in oncology-nonparametric methods. In: Ting, N. (ed.) Dose Finding in Drug Development, 1st edn, pp. 49–58. Springer, New York, NY (2006a)

Ivanova, A.: Escalation, group and $A + B$ designs for dose-finding trials. Stat. Med. **25**(21), 3668–3678 (2006b)

Ivanova, A., Flournoy, N.: Comparison of isotonic designs for dose-finding. Stat. Biopharm. Res. **1**(1), 101–107 (2009)

Ivanova, A., Flournoy, N., Chung, Y.: Cumulative cohort design for dose-finding. J. Stat. Plan. Inference **137**(7), 2316–2327 (2007)

Ivanova, A., Wang, K.: Bivariate isotonic design for dose-finding with ordered groups. Stat. Med. **25**(12), 2018–2026 (2006)

Ivanova, A., Montazer-Haghighi, A., Mohanty, S.G., Durham, S.D.: Improved up-and-down designs for phase I trials. Stat. Med. **22**(1), 69–82 (2003)

Jia, N., Braun, T.M.: The adaptive accelerated biased coin design for phase I clinical trials. J. Appl. Stat. **38**(12), 2911–2924 (2011)

Korn, E.L., Midthune, D., Chen, T.T., Rubinstein, L.V., Christian, M.C., Simon, R.M.: A comparison of two phase I trial designs. Stat. Med. **13**(18), 1799–1806 (1994)

Le Tourneau, C., Lee, J.J., Siu, L.L.: Dose escalation methods in phase I cancer clin. trials. J. Nat. Cancer. Inst. **101**(10), 708–720 (2009)

Leung, D.H.-Y., Wang, Y.-G.: Isotonic designs for phase I trials. Control. Clin. Trials **22**(2), 126–138 (2001)

Leung, D., Wang, Y.-G.: An extension of the continual reassessment method using decision theory. Stat. Med. **21**(1), 51–63 (2002)

Lin, Y., Shih, W.J.: Statistical properties of the traditional algorithm-based designs for phase I cancer clinical trials. Biostatistics **2**(2), 203–215 (2001)

Newell, D.R.: Pharmacologically based phase I trials in cancer chemotherapy. Hematol. Oncol. Clin. North Am. **8**(2), 257–275 (1994)

O'Quigley, J.: Commentary on 'Designs for dose-escalation trials with quantitative responses'. Stat. Med. **28**(30), 3745–3750; 3759–3760 (2009)

Paoletti, X., Ezzalfani, M., Le Tourneau, C.: Statistical controversies in clinical research: requiem for the 3 + 3 design for phase I trials. Ann. Oncol. **26**(9), 1808–1812 (2015)

Paul, R.K., Rosenberger, W.F., Flournoy, N.: Quantile estimation following non-parametric phase I clinical trials with ordinal response. Stat. Med. **23**(16), 2483–2495 (2004)

Ratain, M.J., Mick, R., Schilsky, R.L., Siegler, M.: Statistical and ethical issues in the design and conduct of phase I and II clinical trials of new anticancer agents. J. Nat. Cancer. Inst. **85**(20), 1637–1643 (1993)

Reiner, E., Paoletti, X., O'Quigley, J.: Operating characteristics of the standard phase I clinical trial design. Comput. Stat. Data Anal. **30**(3), 303–315 (1999)

Robertson, T., Wright, F.T., Dykstra, R.: Order Restricted Statistical Inference, 1st edn. John Wiley & Sons, Chichester (1988)

Robbins, H., Monro, S.: A stochastic approximation method. Ann. Math. Stat. **22**(3), 400–407 (1951)

Rogatko, A., Schoeneck, D., Jonas, W., Tighiouart, M., Khuri, F.R., Porter, A.: Translation of innovative designs into phase I trials. J. Clin. Oncol. **25**(31), 4982–4986 (2007)

Rosenberger, W.F., Haines, L.M.: Competing designs for phase I clinical trials: a review. Stat. Med. **21**(18), 2757–2770 (2002)

Sheiner, L.B., Beal, S.L., Sambol, N.C.: Study designs for dose-ranging. Clin. Pharmacol. Ther. **46**(1), 63–77 (1989)

Sheiner, L.B., Hashimoto, Y., Beal, S.L.: A simulation study comparing designs for dose ranging. Stat. Med. **10**(3), 303–321 (1991)

Simon, R.M., Freidlin, B., Rubinstein, L.V., Arbuck, S., Collins, J., Christian, M.: Accelerated titration designs for phase I clinical trials in oncology. J. Nat. Cancer Inst. **89**(15), 1138–47 (1997)

Simon, R., Korn, E.L.: Selecting drug combinations based on total equivalent dose (dose intensity). J. Nat. Cancer Inst. **82**(18), 1469–1476 (1990)

Skolnik, J.M., Barrett, J.S., Jayaraman, B., Patel, D., Adamson, P.C.: Shortening the timeline of pediatric phase I trials: the rolling six design. J. Clin. Oncol. **26**(2), 190–195 (2008)

Smith, T.L., Lee, J.J., Kantarjian, H.M., Legha, S.S., Raber, M.N.: Design and results of phase I cancer clinical trials: three year experience at M.D. Anderson Cancer Center. J. Clin. Oncol. **14**(1), 287–295 (1996)

Storer, B.E.: Design and analysis of phase I clinical trials. Biometrics **45**(3), 925–937 (1989)

Storer, B.E.: Small-sample confidence sets for the MTD in a phase I clinical trial. Biometrics **49**(4), 1117–1125 (1993)

Storer, B.E.: An evaluation of phase I clinical trial designs in the continuous dose-response setting. Stat. Med. **20**(16), 2399–2408 (2001)

Stylianou, M., Flournoy, N.: Dose finding using the biased coin up-and-down design and isotonic regression. Biometrics **58**(1), 171–177 (2002)

Stylianou, M., Follmann, D.A.: The accelerated biased coin up-and-down design in phase I trials. J. Biopharm. Stat. **14**(1), 249–260 (2004)

Stylianou, M., Proschan, M., Flournoy, N.: Estimating the probability of toxicity at the target dose following an up-and-down design. Stat. Med. **22**(4), 535–543 (2003)

Tsutakawa, R.K.: Random walk design in bio-assay. J. Am. Stat. Assoc. **62**(319), 842–856 (1967a)

Tsutakawa, R.K.: Asymptotic properties of the block up-and-down method in bio-assay. Ann. Math. Stat. **38**(6), 1822–1828 (1967b)

von Békésy, G.: A new audiometer. Acta Otolaryngol. **35**(5–6), 411–422 (1947)

Wetherill, G.B.: Sequential estimation of quantal response curves. J. R. Stat. Soc.: Series B **25**(1), 1–48 (1963)

Wetherill, G.B., Levitt, H.: Sequential estimation of points on a psychometric function. Brit. J. Math. Stat. Psy. **18**(1), 1–10 (1965)

Wheeler, G.M., Sweeting, M.J., Mander, A.P.: AplusB: a web application for investigating A + B designs for phase I cancer clinical trials. PLoS ONE **11**(7), e0159026 (2016)

Wu, C.: Efficient sequential designs with binary data. J. Am. Stat. Assoc. **80**(392), 974–984 (1985)

Yuan, Z., Chappell, R.: Isotonic designs for phase I cancer clinical trials with multiple risk groups. Clin. Trials **1**(6), 499–508 (2004)

Zohar, S., O'Quigley, J.: Re: Dose escalation methods in phase I cancer clinical trials. J. Nat. Cancer Inst. **101**(24), 1732–1733 (2009)

Chapter 3
Model-Based Designs Considering Toxicity Alone

Abstract Phase I trial designs in oncology aim to determine the maximum tolerated doses for agents of interest. Traditionally, dose-finding designs for phase I trials can be classified as rule-/algorithm- or model-based designs. In Chap. 2, we focused on rule-based designs; in the present chapter, we focus on model-based designs. Model-based designs assume a certain statistical model for the monotonic dose–toxicity relationship to borrow strength across doses, and originate from the continual reassessment method (CRM). The present chapter provides a detailed description of the concepts, theories, properties, and advantages and disadvantages of the CRM, and also overview designs that are related to the CRM or that constitute extended versions of this method.

Keywords Maximum tolerated dose (MTD) · Model-based designs · Continual reassessment method (CRM)

3.1 Introduction

The standard-bearer of model-based designs is the continual reassessment method (CRM), which was proposed by O'Quigley et al. (1990). Since this method was first proposed, numerous modified or expanded versions and related designs have been developed to overcome various problems that arise during practical application of the CRM. Therefore, in this chapter, we first describe the basic concepts, theories, properties, and advantages and disadvantages of the CRM in detail; then, we overview various model-based designs.

Unless specifically noted, suppose that the aim of a phase I trial with a prespecified maximum sample size is to identify the maximum tolerated dose (MTD) of an agent among increasing ordered doses $d_1 < \ldots < d_K$ corresponding to $1, \ldots, K$ dose levels, which are prespecified using the modified Fibonacci or other methods in a manner that includes the true MTD (see, e.g., Collins et al. 1986, Edler and Burkholder 2006).

3.2   Continual Reassessment Method

3.2.1 Notation and Requirements

Let X_j ($j = 1, \ldots, n$) denote the random variable for the dose administered to
the jth patient enrolled in the trial, and let x_j represent an observed value. Because
K fixed doses $\{d_1, \ldots, d_K\}$ are usually available, x_j has some discrete value: $x_j \in$
$\{d_1, \ldots, d_K\}$. If not, it has some continuous value within a positive real-valued space
$x_j \in \mathfrak{R}^+$. Let Y_j ($j = 1, \ldots, n$) denote the binary random variable for a toxic
response of the jth patient, and let y_j indicate an observed value. Then, y_j is equal
to 1 if the jth patient experiences a toxic response or to 0 otherwise. Let $R(x) =$
$\Pr(Y_j = 1 | X = x)$ denote the true toxicity probability at dose x for the jth patient,
which is assumed to be an expectation of Y_j given $X = d_k$ ($k = 1, \ldots, K$), that is,
$R(x) = \Pr(Y_j = 1 | X = x) = \mathrm{E}(Y_j | X = x)$. We consider a simple dose–toxicity
function for $\mathrm{E}(Y_j | X = x)$ and denote it by $\psi(x, \beta)$, where β is a variable defined
in set $\mathfrak{B}$. Consequently, we obtain the following model for the relationship between
$R(x)$ and $\psi(x, \beta)$:

$$R(x) = \Pr(Y_j = 1 | X = x) = \mathrm{E}(Y_j | X = x) = \psi(x, \beta). \tag{3.1}$$

Note that, under this statistical model, β is no longer a variable but an unknown
parameter to be estimated.

The function $\psi(x, \beta)$ has the following requirements:

1. For a given fixed value of x, this function is strictly monotonic in β, and for a
   fixed value of β, it is monotonically increasing in x.
2. For discrete doses d_k, the values of $\psi(d_k, \beta)$ only must be ordered; thus, the
   values of d_k need not be ordered. Therefore, we must only note the "level" k of
   dose d_k. That is, whenever $k > k'$, $\psi(d_k, \beta) > \psi(d_{k'}, \beta)$.
3. For doses d_k, there exist values of β, say $\beta_1, \ldots, \beta_K \in \mathfrak{B}$, such that $R(d_k) =$
   $\psi(d_k, \beta_k)$ ($k = 1, \ldots, K$). In other words, this single-parameter model must be
   sufficiently rich to model the true toxicity probability at any dose level.

Requirement 1 indicates that there is a dose x^* that yields $\psi(x^*, \beta_0) = \Gamma_{\mathrm{T}}$ for a
given value β_0 of β, where Γ_{T} is any target toxicity probability level. Furthermore, for
any x^* and Γ_{T}, there is a single value β^* that satisfies $\psi(x^*, \beta^*) = \Gamma_{\mathrm{T}}$. Requirement
2 indicates that, if the correspondence between k and d_k is established, it is possible
to express x as $x \in \{1, \ldots, K\}$. This is indicative of k being available as a label for the
dose set, provided script d is ignored and attention is paid to k only. In a sense, d_k is
only the conceptual dose and need not be the dose that is actually used. Requirement
3 indicates that the model represented by Eq. (3.1) is sufficiently flexible to represent
the true toxicity probability at a given dose level (particularly at or near the MTD).
However, in reality, model (3.1) cannot usually be correctly assumed, that is, it cannot
be anticipated that $\beta_1 = \ldots = \beta_K = \beta$. Therefore, this model is called a "working
model."

Suppose that the MTD exists and is denoted by d_0, and d_0 is estimated as one of the available doses $\{d_1, \ldots, d_K\}$: $d_0 \in \{d_1, \ldots, d_K\}$. Therefore, d_0 satisfies

$$\Delta(R(d_0), \Gamma_T) < \Delta(R(d_k), \Gamma_T), \ k = 1, \ldots, K; \ d_k \neq d_0, \tag{3.2}$$

where $\Delta(R(d_0), \Gamma_T)$ is some measure of distance between $R(d_0)$ and Γ_T. For example, $\Delta(R(d_0), \Gamma_T) = \|R(d_0) - \Gamma_T\|$, and $\Delta(R(d_0), \Gamma_T) = (R(d_0) - \Gamma_T)^2$.

3.2.2 Working Models

There are many possible candidates for the working model $\psi(x, \beta)$. For example, O'Quigley et al. (1990) proposed the following hyperbolic tangent model, because the hyperbolic tangent function $\tanh(x)$ increases monotonically from 0 to 1 as x increases from $-\infty$ to ∞:

$$\psi(x, \beta) = [\{\tanh(x) + 1\}/2]^\beta, \tag{3.3}$$

where $0 < \beta < \infty$. In particular, when $x \in \{d_1, \ldots, d_K\}$ and provided the working model (3.3) can be replaced with $a_k = \{\tanh(d_k) + 1\}/2$ for $k = 1, \ldots, K$ (in other words, the dose level d_K is recoded), the result is equivalent to a power model or empirical model expressed as

$$\psi(d_k, \beta) = a_k^\beta, \tag{3.4}$$

where $0 < a_1 < \ldots < a_K < 1$. The working model (3.4) can be rewritten through parameterization as $\psi(d_k, \beta) = a_k^{\exp(\beta)}$ for $k = 1, \ldots, K$, and support for parameter β can be expanded to the whole real line, where $-\infty < \beta < \infty$.

Here, as stated above, it should be noted that the d_k (or the recoded a_k) prespecified during trial planning is not the actually administered dose. Instead, it is the conceptual dose obtained by back-substituting an initial guess for the toxicity probability at each dose level into the working model (see Garrett-Mayer 2006). For example, if six doses can be used in a given trial, suppose that the following toxicity probabilities across low to high doses are guessed prior to the start of the trial: 0.05, 0.10, 0.20, 0.30, 0.50, and 0.70, respectively. Here, if working model (3.3) is used, β is fixed at a certain value, say 1, and the conceptual doses are set to $d_1 = -1.47$, $d_2 = -1.10$, $d_3 = -0.69$, $d_4 = -0.42$, $d_5 = 0.0$, and $d_6 = 0.42$. These conceptual doses do not directly represent the actual available doses, but indirectly correspond to them. On the other hand, if working model (3.4) is used, $a_1 = 0.05$, $a_2 = 0.10$, $a_3 = 0.20$, $a_4 = 0.30$, $a_5 = 0.50$, and $a_6 = 0.70$ are set. Although the two sets of guesses differ with regard to the working model, the guesses for the toxicity probability at each dose level are equivalent. Consequently, a_k ($k = 1, \ldots, K$) is sometimes called "initial guess" (for the probability of toxicity) or "skeleton." If a likelihood-based estimation method (see Sect. 3.2.2.2) is adopted, use of working model (3.4) becomes equivalent to use of a working model that replaces a_k with a_k^* satisfying $a_k^* = a_k^r$ ($k = 1, \ldots, K$) for any positive real value $r > 0$ in estimation of parameter β. Thus, no interpretation of a_k is possible. Consequently, although it is common to conflate the two aforementioned names: "initial guess" and "skeleton", if a rigorous distinction is to be made, the former is associated with use in Bayesian inferential procedures (see Sect. 3.2.2.1), while the latter is associated with use in likelihood-based estimation procedures (see Sect. 3.2.2.2). In addition, the spacing between neighboring values of a_k (or d_k) is decided so as to reflect the initially guessed toxicity probability. It should be noted that this naturally affects the CRM operating characteristics. Lee and Cheung (2009) have suggested a systematic method for determination of this spacing.

It is also possible to consider working models different from those discussed above. For example, the following fixed-intercept, one-parameter logistic model can be considered:

$$\psi(d_k, \beta) = \frac{\exp(b_c + \beta d_k)}{1 + \exp(b_c + \beta d_k)}, \tag{3.5}$$

or the following fixed-slope, one-parameter logistic model:

$$\psi(d_k, \beta) = \frac{\exp(\beta + b_c d_k)}{1 + \exp(\beta + b_c d_k)}, \tag{3.6}$$

where b_c is a fixed value. If further flexibility is sought, another possibility is a two-parameter logistic model that regards b_c as a parameter in working model (3.6):

$$\psi(d_k, \beta_1, \beta_2) = \frac{\exp(\beta_1 + \beta_2 d_k)}{1 + \exp(\beta_1 + \beta_2 d_k)}. \tag{3.7}$$

The candidate doses in a phase I trial are often determined by the modified Fibonacci method (for example, if $d_1 = 1$ in the modified Fibonacci method, the subsequent doses are $d_2 = 2$, $d_3 = 3$, $d_4 = 4.5$, $d_5 = 6$, and $d_6 = 8$). However, by noting the dose increment between two adjacent dose levels in a dose sequence, the working model can be adapted to some extent (Paoletti and Kramar 2009). For example, working models (3.3) and (3.4) are suitable for sequences in which the absolute increment ($d_{k+1} - d_k$) is constant, whereas working model (3.5) is suitable for sequences in which the relative increment (($d_{k+1} - d_k)/d_k$) is constant. In particular, as regards the odds ratio of the risk between two adjacent dose levels in working models (3.5) and (3.6), the dose increment is proportional to $\exp((d_{k+1} - d_k)/d_k)$ in working model (3.5) and proportional to $\exp(d_{k+1} - d_k)$ in working model (3.6). If the number of dose levels is not particularly high, the relative and absolute increases are both approximately constant. However, if there are many dose levels, attention must be paid to the increment when selecting the working model. In this regard, the dose increment obtained using the modified Fibonacci method is an intermediate value between the absolute and relative increments and, in any case, can be roughly considered constant. Thus, either working model (3.3) or (3.5) may be justifiably used for doses determined by the modified Fibonacci method.

According to Shen and O'Quigley (1996), even if the working model is misspecified, including the case of incorrect spacing, the dose recommended by the CRM under a certain condition asymptotically converges to the true MTD. This indicates that the working model is also sufficiently robust in such a scenario (see Sect. 3.2.3). However, as the number of subjects in phase I trials is generally limited to only tens of patients, and although the choice of working model does not strongly influence the CRM operating characteristics (Chevret 1993), this choice is still somewhat relevant (Paoletti and Kramar 2009). As regards, the working model that should be used, O'Quigley et al. (1990), who proposed the CRM, assert that a one-parameter model is sufficient (for example, see Shen and O'Quigley 1996 and O'Quigley 2006a), other than for some specialized cases (see, e.g., O'Quigley and Paoletti 2003). Paoletti and Kramar (2009) focused primarily on the Bayesian CRM (see Sect. 3.2.2.1) and evaluated the influence of the choice of working model (one- versus two-parameter models), on the spacing between dose levels in a power model. They also considered the effects of many dose levels before the MTD is reached, from the perspective of the efficiency of the nonparametric optimal design given by O'Quigley et al. (2002). In their work, Paoletti and Kramar (2009) used the design presented by Paoletti et al. (2004) as an evaluation tool for the CRM operating characteristics. Paoletti and Kramar (2009) reported the following:

- A one-parameter power model has superior performance to a two-parameter logistic model.
- Although there is no method for optimally attaining the spacing between dose levels for all scenarios in the power model, that used by Shen and O'Quigley (1996) yields favorable performance.
- If many dose levels exist before the MTD is reached, a two-parameter logistic model is useful; however, a well-calibrated power model can also be useful.
- A Bayesian estimation method (for example, see Gatsonis and Greenhouse 1992 and Whitehead and Williamson 1998) may be effective for resolving the problem of parameter non-identification in a two-parameter logistic model (for example, see Shu and O'Quigley 2008).

3.2.2.1 Bayesian CRM

Let $\mathcal{D}_j = \{(x_1, y_1), \ldots, (x_{j-1}, y_{j-1})\}$ $(j = 1, \ldots, n)$ denote data consisting of administered dose pairs and toxic responses up to the $(j - 1)$th patient enrolled in the trial, and $p(\beta, \mathcal{D}_j)$ $(j = 1, \ldots, n)$ denote a posterior distribution of parameter β when $\mathcal{D}_j$ has been obtained. Thus, this posterior distribution serves as a prior distribution before dose assignment and toxicity evaluation with respect to the jth patient. Because $p(\beta, \mathcal{D}_j)$ is a nonnegative function representing available prior information on the value of β and information on $\mathcal{D}_j$, it satisfies

$$\int_{\beta \in \mathfrak{B}} p(\beta, \mathfrak{D}_j) \mathrm{d}\beta = 1.$$

The Bayesian estimate $\tilde{\beta}$ of β is given by the posterior expected value of β:

$$\tilde{\beta} = \int_{\beta \in \mathfrak{B}} \beta p(\beta, \mathfrak{D}_j) \mathrm{d}\beta. \tag{3.8}$$

The Bayesian estimate $\tilde{R}(d_k)$ of $R(d_k)$ at dose level k is given by the posterior expected value of the toxicity probability based on $\mathfrak{D}_j$:

$$\tilde{R}(d_k) = \int_{\beta \in \mathfrak{B}} \psi(d_k, \beta) p(\beta, \mathfrak{D}_j) \mathrm{d}\beta. \tag{3.9}$$

As apparent from Eq. (3.9), K integrals are required. Note that O'Quigley et al. (1990) used $\tilde{R}(d_k) = \psi(d_k, \tilde{\beta})$, for $k = 1, \ldots, K$, as an alternative estimate for $\tilde{R}(d_k)$ so as to reduce the K integrals to one integral (considering the limitations of the computing environment at the time). However, the approach based on Eq. (3.9) is more direct (Ishizuka and Ohashi 2001) and favorable when large numbers of patients are enrolled in the trials (Chu et al. 2009). O'Quigley et al. (1990) and O'Quigley (1992) presented an analytical solution for calculating the integral in Eq. (3.9); however, the difference in the calculation results given by the analytical and numerical solutions is not particularly large (Bensadon and O'Quigley 1994).

In the CRM, the dose x_j assigned to the newly enrolled jth patient with the purpose of administering it as the MTD is the dose satisfying the following equation:

$$\Delta(\tilde{R}(x_j), \Gamma_T) < \Delta(\tilde{R}(d_k), \Gamma_T), \quad k = 1, \ldots, K; \ d_k \neq x_j, \tag{3.10}$$

where Γ_T is the target toxicity probability level.

As apparent from comparison of Eqs. (3.10) to (3.2), the overall goal of MTD estimation in a dose-finding trial accords with the specific goal of treating individual patients with the MTD. This can be considered a major advantage of the CRM. In Eq. (3.10), $\Delta(\tilde{R}(x_j), \Gamma_T)$ can be replaced with $\Delta(\tilde{R}(x_j), \Gamma_T)$ or $\Delta(x_j, \psi^{-1}_{\beta = \tilde{\beta}}(\Gamma_T))$, which is the distance measure. In addition, instead of using this distance measure, the dose to be administered can be determined using the probability of controlling the overdose likelihood (Babb et al. 1998) or by using a gain function regarding the precision of the MTD estimation for the next enrolled patient (Whitehead and Brunier 1995). Neuenschwander et al. (2008) developed a method of dose administration that maximizes the posterior probability that the toxicity will fall within a target range. This method is called the Bayesian logistic regression method (BLRM). Furthermore, random assignment of a dose level that is one above or below the level recommended by Eq. (3.10) to the next enrolled patient is also an option, which could solve the problem of parameter non-identifiability that arises in the two-parameter model (for example, see Shu and O'Quigley 2008, O'Quigley 2006a, O'Quigley and Conaway 2010).

When the jth enrolled patient is treated with dose x_j and the toxicity evaluation for that patient yields the result y_j, Bayes' theorem can be used to obtain $p(\beta, \mathfrak{D}_{j+1})$ from $p(\beta, \mathfrak{D}_j)$, which updates the information regarding the value of parameter β_0. That is,

$$
\begin{aligned}
p(\beta, \mathfrak{D}_{j+1}) &= \frac{\{\psi(x_j, \beta)\}^{y_j}\{1 - \psi(x_j, \beta)\}^{(1-y_j)} p(\beta, \mathfrak{D}_j)}{\displaystyle\int_{-\infty}^{\infty}\{\psi(x_j, \beta)\}^{y_j}\{1 - \psi(x_j, \beta)\}^{(1-y_j)} p(\beta, \mathfrak{D}_j)\mathrm{d}\beta} \\
&= \frac{\mathfrak{L}_j(\beta)g(\beta)}{\displaystyle\int_{-\infty}^{\infty}\mathfrak{L}_j(\beta)g(\beta)\mathrm{d}\beta},
\end{aligned} \tag{3.11}
$$

where $\mathfrak{L}_j(\beta)$ is the likelihood function of β, given by

$$
\mathfrak{L}_j(\beta) = \prod_{l=1}^{j}\{\psi(x_l, \beta)\}^{y_l}\{1 - \psi(x_l, \beta)\}^{(1-y_l)}. \tag{3.12}
$$

In addition, $g(\beta)$ is defined as $g(\beta) = p(\beta, \mathfrak{D}_1)$ and constitutes the prior distribution of β, reflecting information regarding the relationship between the dose and toxicity that should be known prior to the start of the trial. Consequently, the dose assigned to the next (i.e., $(j + 1)$th) enrolled patient is determined via Eq. (3.10) using $p(\beta, \mathfrak{D}_{j+1})$, as described above.

In the CRM, each time a new patient is enrolled, a continual reassessment is performed using data on the doses that have already been administered to previously enrolled patients and any observed toxic responses. Hence, a recommendation is made for treatment of the newly enrolled patients as per the best estimate for the MTD at the given point in time. However, the dose assigned using the CRM may be, at best, a recommendation and is not mandatory. Instead, the dose determined by a clinician after comprehensive consideration of a patient's specific toxicity status (such as the dose-limiting toxicity (DLT) or other toxicity); the results of a pharmacokinetic evaluation; or the opinions of an independent Data Monitoring Committee, an Efficacy and Safety Evaluation Committee, etc., could be prioritized (Paoletti et al. 2006). Ultimately, if the maximum number of patients enrolled in a trial is fixed at n and the trial is not suspended early (before n is reached), the MTD is determined as the dose that can treat a hypothetical patient (i.e., one not actually enrolled) as the $(n + 1)$th patient. The toxicity should be evaluated and recorded cautiously, because errors in toxicity data influence the MTD determination. This is particularly true when toxicity is erroneously considered to be present (Zohar and O'Quigley 2009).

In addition, there are cases in which the CRM is not used to estimate the MTD of an anticancer agent, but rather to search for the minimum effective dose of a generic agent (see Resche-Rigon et al. 2008 and Zohar et al. 2013).

When implementing a Bayesian CRM as described above, one major concern is selection of $g(\beta)$, because of its dependence on the Bayesian inference. One natural candidate for $g(\beta)$ is the gamma prior distribution for $\beta = (0, \infty)$ (Onar et al. 2009):

$$g(\beta) = v_1^{v_2} \beta^{v_2-1} \exp(-v_1\beta),$$

where v_1 is a scale parameter and v_2 is a shape parameter. In particular, if $v_1 = v_2 = 1$, the exponential distribution has a mean of 1. Under relatively simple circumstances in which the number of dose levels is not particularly large, this exponential prior distribution approach can give satisfactory results from the perspective of its operating characteristics (Onar et al. 2009); however, this is not always the case (Møller 1995). It is possible to assume a parametric density function, but it is also possible to indirectly specify $g(\beta)$ using pseudo-data, instead of directly specifying the functional form of $g(\beta)$ (O'Quigley and Conaway 2010). If y_l^* ($l = 1, .., n_{\text{pseudo}}$) denote the pseudo-data, $g(\beta)$ is specified as

$$g(\beta) \approx \exp\left[\sum_{l=1}^{n^{\text{pseudo}}} y_l^* \log \psi(x_l, \beta) + \sum_{l=1}^{n^{\text{pseudo}}} (1 - y_l^*) \log(1 - \psi(x_l, \beta))\right]. \quad (3.13)$$

The right-hand side of Eq. (3.13) takes the same form as the result obtained from exponentiation following application of the logarithm of likelihood in Eq. (3.12). Consequently, if this form is used as an intermediary, it is possible to calculate the posterior distribution without calculating the integral by adding the obtained data, even if a software package with no Bayesian calculations is used (see, e.g., Whitehead and Brunier 1995 and Murphy and Hall 1997). In a study by Whitehead and Brunier (1995), a prior distribution based on such pseudo-data was utilized to construct a beta prior distribution of the parameters in a two-parameter logistic model. Murphy and Hall (1997) also discussed a dose-finding design that utilized a prior distribution based on pseudo-data (called a "seed" in their paper).

In addition, it is also possible to obtain a posterior distribution by considering the uncertainty of a prior distribution on the basis of the pseudo-data and the data that has been actually obtained. Specifically, if we combine the prior distribution obtained from the pseudo-data with the likelihood calculated from the actually obtained data by means of the weighting coefficient $w_j, 0 < w_j < 1$ ($j = 1, \ldots, n$), the following posterior density function can be obtained (O'Quigley and Conaway 2010):

$$p(\beta, \mathfrak{D}_{j+1}) = W_j^{-1} \exp\left\{w_j \log g(\beta) + (1 - w_j)\mathfrak{L}_j(\beta)\right\}, \quad (3.14)$$

where $W_j = \int_{\beta \in \mathfrak{B}} \exp\left\{w_j \log g(\beta) + (1 - w_j)\mathfrak{L}_j(\beta)\right\} d\beta$. Note that w_j must ordinarily be set such that $w_j < w_{j-1}$ if it is to be dependent on j. However, in many actual circumstances, there is no need for dependence on j; thus, it is acceptable for w_j to be a sufficiently small constant that does not unnecessarily affect the prior distribution estimated from the pseudo-data.

Instead of the pseudo-data, it is also possible to use preliminary trial data as-is (see, e.g., Piantadosi et al. 1998 and Legedza and Ibrahim 2001). Alternatively, a prior distribution can be constructed based on the perceptions of clinicians regarding the results (see Morita 2011). In such cases, the prior distribution is an informative prior because it actively uses information from preliminary trials. O'Quigley (2006a) suggested a method of constructing informative and noninformative priors as per the dose levels by dividing the intervals for β by the number of dose levels and applying probability masses to each. Incorporation of an informative prior can be desirable depending on the trial, but it must not override the data observed after the trial has been initiated, unlike the case of noninformative priors. In this context, Morita (2011) presented examples of application of informative priors to clinical trials in practice and introduced methods to quantify these priors and to investigate their appropriateness using the prior effective sample size (Morita et al. 2008). Furthermore, Takeda and Morita (2018) considered incorporating historical data from a previous trial to design and conduct a subsequent trial in a different patient population. In addition, Asakawa et al. (2012) presented a design that adaptively changes the prior distribution based on the toxicity evaluation results obtained for a cohort to which the starting dose is administered.

3.2.2.2   Likelihood-Based CRM

The original CRM proposed by O'Quigley et al. (1990) is based on a Bayesian framework as, discussed above. However, this aspect yields some difficulties, which are as follows:

- Even if vague and insufficient information is used, or even if patient data regarding dose assignment and toxicity have a diminished impact, a prior distribution, which is often the target of criticism from non-Bayesian scholars, must be used.
- Usually, if a parametric prior distribution is assumed, it is not conjugated; accordingly, a numerical integral calculation is required in such cases.
- In the CRM, unlike other designs (e.g., those reported by Storer 1989), the dose administered to the initial patient enrolled in the trial (in other words, the starting dose) is determined based on the prior distribution. This is because the data are naturally not yet accumulated at that time. Therefore, the administered dose is not necessarily the lowest dose and thus may be unsafe.

One solution for the first and second difficulties is to base the estimation method in the CRM on the likelihood. However, to utilize a likelihood-based estimation method, it is necessary to prevent the parameter estimate from lying at the boundaries between the parameter spaces and to ensure that the likelihood is not monotonic. This requires heterogeneity of the toxicity between patients; in other words, the presence and absence of toxicity must be observed in at least one patient, respectively

(Silvapulle 1981). If such heterogeneity is not observed, the likelihood will reach its maximum value at the boundaries between the parameter spaces; the estimate of $R(d_k)$ $(k = 1, ..., K)$ will become 0 or 1; and the estimate will not be definable based on the working model. This scenario can also be regarded as a new difficulty that arises when a likelihood-based estimation method is employed in conjunction with sequential patient enrollment, and when the presence and absence of toxicity among them cannot necessarily be expected to be heterogenic.

O'Quigley and Shen (1996) developed a likelihood-based CRM for resolving the three difficulties noted above, as well as the difficulties that arise when a likelihood-based estimation method is adopted. The likelihood-based CRM utilizes the benefit of the two-stage design developed by Storer (1989). This approach allows for quick arrival at the MTD through dose escalation until toxicity is observed early in the first stage; in such trials, a low dose that may not have a therapeutic effect may otherwise be used. Consequently, while maintaining the aim of the first stage, this design enables achievement of heterogeneity in the presence or absence of toxicity among patients, as required by likelihood-based estimation.

The dose-finding algorithm of the likelihood-based CRM is as follows:

- Stage 1: Start the trial by administering the lowest dose to a cohort comprising a single patient or multiple patients. Then, until heterogeneity of toxicity is observed, use a dose escalation design or Bayesian CRM to assign doses to an individual patient or cohort, followed by toxicity evaluation. Go to Stage 2.
- Stage 2: Conduct the dose assignment and MTD estimation based on the maximum likelihood estimates obtained by maximizing the likelihood in the likelihood-based CRM.

Because dose finding is performed using the above two stages, the likelihood-based CRM is sometimes referred to as "two-stage CRM" or by a name (i.e., "two-stage design," see Sect. 2.4) similar to that of the design proposed by Storer (1989). Prior to O'Quigley and Shen (1996), Møller (1995) presented the same design, but with a Bayesian CRM framework, which only inherited the abovementioned concept from Storer (1989).

To describe the second stage of the likelihood-based CRM in more detail, for which data are acquired for patients up to the jth patient, the logarithm of the likelihood function is presented as follows:

$$\log \mathcal{L}_j(\beta) = \sum_{l=1}^{j} y_l \log \psi(x_l, \beta) + \sum_{l=1}^{j} (1 - y_l) \log(1 - \psi(x_l, \beta)). \qquad (3.15)$$

The maximum likelihood estimate $\hat{\beta}$ of β is obtained by maximizing Eq. (3.15). The probability of toxicity is estimated using the $\hat{\beta}$ in $\hat{R}(d_k) = \psi(d_k, \hat{\beta})$ $(k = 1, \ldots, K)$. As a result, it is possible to assign doses and estimate the MTD, similar to when a Bayesian CRM is used.

In the likelihood-based CRM, the prior distribution for β is not prespecified, of course; however, the data obtained up to the end of the first stage can be regarded as an empirical prior. In this sense, it is possible to reconsider the entirety of the Bayesian framework, while retaining the original characteristics of the sequential learning process in the Bayesian CRM. A revised version of the design developed by Murphy and Hall (1997) that exploits this two-stage design concept has been presented by Wang and Faries (2000).

3.2.2.3 Credible and Confidence Intervals for Toxicity Probability

The methods for estimating the credible and confidence intervals for the toxicity probability and the parameters of the working model specified in the CRM differ depending on whether Bayesian- or likelihood-based inference are used, as indicated in the previous section. O'Quigley (1992) introduced a method to estimate the two intervals for the toxicity probability and working model parameters after data have been obtained for the final (nth) registered patient. For example, if the likelihood-based estimation method is used, the $100(1-a)\%$ confidence interval (ψ_n^L, ψ_n^U) for the toxicity probability $\psi(x_{n+1}, \hat{\beta}_n)$ given parameter estimate $\hat{\beta}_n$ can be constructed as

$$\psi_n^L = \psi\left\{x_{n+1}, (\hat{\beta}_n + z_{1-\alpha/2}\widehat{\mathrm{Var}}(\hat{\beta}_n)^{1/2})\right\}, \ \psi_n^U = \psi\left\{x_{n+1}, (\hat{\beta}_n - z_{1-\alpha/2}\widehat{\mathrm{Var}}(\hat{\beta}_n)^{1/2})\right\},$$

(3.16)

where $z_{1-\alpha/2}$ is the $100(1-\alpha/2)$ percent point of the standard normal distribution and $\widehat{\mathrm{Var}}(\hat{\beta}_n)$ represents the estimate of the variance of $\hat{\beta}_n$. Note that the working model can always be misspecified, because the true relationship between the dose and toxicity is unknown. However, regardless of whether a Bayesian- or likelihood-based approach is used, the constructed confidence or credible intervals are useful in practice, because the coverage probability is close to the nominal level. This holds even if the sample size is small (12–20) (O'Quigley 1992; Natarajan and O'Quigley 2003). In particular, if an exponential distribution is used as the prior distribution in a Bayesian approach, favorable performance is obtained by using a Cornish–Fisher approximation for construction of the credible interval. Note that Iasonos and Ostrovnaya (2011) proposed a method based on a constrained maximum likelihood method as another means of constructing the confidence interval.

3.2.3 Convergence

One of the attractive characteristics of the CRM is that the doses it recommends eventually converge to the true MTD. This argument is based on the use of a likelihood-based CRM but, provided the prior distribution does not degenerate, it is also applicable to a Bayesian CRM. However, because the working model in the CRM is misspecified, it collapses in a usual likelihood argument. Nevertheless, as indicated in Sect. 3.2.2.2, β is estimated by maximizing Eq. (3.12) or (3.15). This is equivalent to determining the derivative function of Eq. (3.15), setting the right-hand side to zero, and then solving the resulting estimating equation. To investigate the phenomenon of convergence in the context of MTD determination after dose assignment and toxicity evaluation have been completed for the final (nth) enrolled patient, Shen and O'Quigley (1996) defined this process as follows:

$$U_n(\beta) = \frac{1}{n} \sum_{j=1}^{n} \left[y_j \frac{\psi'}{\psi} \{x_j, \beta\} + (1 - y_j) \frac{-\psi'}{1 - \psi} \{x_j, \beta\} \right], \qquad (3.17)$$

and

$$\tilde{U}_n(\beta) = \frac{1}{n} \sum_{j=1}^{n} \left[R(x_j) \frac{\psi'}{\psi} \{x_j, \beta\} + (1 - R(x_j)) \frac{-\psi'}{1 - \psi} \{x_j, \beta\} \right], \qquad (3.18)$$

where ψ' is the derivative function of $\psi(x_j, \beta)$. Shen and O'Quigley (1996) indicated that, under some conditions, it is *almost surely* $\sup_{\beta \in [B_{\text{lower}}, B_{\text{upper}}]} |U_n(\beta) - \tilde{U}_n(\beta)| \to 0$, where $[B_{\text{lower}}, B_{\text{upper}}]$ is a finite interval in which the value of β exists. As a result, β_n converges to β^*, satisfying $R(d^*) = \psi(d^*, \beta^*) = \Gamma_T^*$, and the asymptotic distribution of $\sqrt{n}(\hat{\beta}_n - \beta^*)$ has a normal distribution with a mean of 0 and variance σ^2, denoted by N(0, σ^2). Here, d^* is the true MTD, Γ_T^* is the true toxicity probability, and $\sigma^2 = \{\psi(d^*, \beta^*)\}^{-2} \Gamma_T^*(1 - \Gamma_T^*)$. Generally, it is expected that $\Gamma_T^* \neq \Gamma_T$, but that their values are close. It has also been shown that, at the same time, x_{n+1} converges to d^* or its neighborhood. (For details, see Shen and O'Quigley 1996 and O'Quigley 2006a.)

3.2.4 Efficiency

It is possible to use $\hat{\Gamma}_{T,n}^* = \psi(x_{n+1}, \hat{\beta}_n)$ to estimate the toxicity probability at the recommended dose, when the dose assignment and toxicity evaluation have been completed for the final (nth) enrolled patient (O'Quigley 1992). If the delta method is applied, the asymptotic distribution of $\sqrt{n}(\hat{\Gamma}_{T,n}^* - R(d^*))$ can be shown to be the normal distribution N(0, $\Gamma_T^*(1 - \Gamma_T^*)$) (Shen and O'Quigley 1996). In other words, this estimate given by the CRM is effective for large sample sizes only. However, the number of patients enrolled in a phase I trial is limited; thus, the efficiency of this estimate must be evaluated on a case-by-case basis using simulations performed under a variety of scenarios and based on this limited number of patients. O'Quigley (1992) studied this issue and indicated that the mean square error of the estimated toxicity probability at the recommended dose is consistent with the theoretical variance. The efficiency obtained for such a limited sample can also be evaluated using the nonparametric optimal design proposed by O'Quigley et al. (2002).

3.2.5 Sensitivity Analysis and Calibration of Working Models

The dose recommended by the CRM is consistent with the MTD or a dose close to it, even if the working model is misspecified (see, e.g., Shen and O'Quigley 1996 and O'Quigley 2006a). Cheung and Chappell (2002) presented the conditions sufficient for this consistency and discussed the methodology for sensitivity evaluation of the working model employed in the CRM (see also, Chevret (1993), as simulations were used to study the CRM sensitivity to the working model specifications and parameter prior distribution in that work).

Suppose the working model is $\psi(d_k, \beta) = \psi_k(\beta)$ $(k = 1, \ldots, K)$. For dose level j with $j = 1, \ldots, K$, we define

$$\mathfrak{B}_j = \{\beta \in \mathcal{B} : |\psi_j(\beta) - \Gamma_T| < |\psi_k(\beta) - \Gamma_T|, k \neq j\}, \qquad (3.19)$$

where the parameter space $\mathfrak{B}$ is assumed to be a closed finite interval $[\beta_1, \beta_{K+1}]$. Then, $\mathfrak{B}_1 = [\beta_1, \beta_2)$, $\mathfrak{B}_k = (\beta_k, \beta_{k+1}]$ $(k = 2, \ldots, K - 1)$, $\mathfrak{B}_K = (\beta_K, \beta_{K+1})$, and β_k is a solution of $\psi_k(\beta_{k-1}) + \psi_k(\beta_k) = 2\Gamma_T$ (Cheung and Chappell 2002; O'Quigley, 2006a). Let $\hat{\beta}_n$ denote the parameter estimate based on the data for the nth patient. The CRM recommends dose level j only when $\hat{\beta}_n \in \mathfrak{B}_j$. Furthermore, letting $\Gamma_{T,k}^*$ denote the true toxicity probability at dose level k, we define $\beta_k^* = \psi_k^{-1}(\Gamma_{T,k}^*)$ (if the working model ψ is correct, $\beta_k = \beta_0$ with respect to some true parameter value β_0 for all k). On this basis, Cheung and Chappell (2002) presented the following two sufficient conditions:

(C1)   For all k, $\beta_k^* \in \mathfrak{B}_l$, where l is the correct dose level corresponding to the true MTD.

(C2) $\beta_l^* \in \mathfrak{B}_l$: for $k = 1, \ldots, l - 1$, $\beta_k^* \in \cup_{j=k+1}^{K} \mathfrak{B}_j$; and for $k = l + 1, \ldots, K$, $\beta_k^* \in \cup_{j=1}^{k-1} \mathfrak{B}_j$.

Given the true toxicity probability and using these sufficient conditions, it is possible to understand (prior to simulation implementation) the sensitivity of the working model from the perspective of convergence of the recommended dose under the prespecified working model to the MTD. It is also possible to determine which working model should be used.

Of course, the true relationship between dose and toxicity remains unknown. In this context, it has been further shown that an indifference interval exists for the toxicity probability for each dose level. In these intervals, the probability of a toxic response at the dose level adjacent to that corresponding to the correct MTD is sufficiently close to Γ_T; thus, the dose level adjacent to the dose level corresponding to the correct MTD is selected in its stead. In other words, the indifference interval is the interval sufficient for clinicians to be indifferent to the difference, even if the MTD is selected as such an incorrect dose level. This indifference interval yields a range that includes the toxicity probability at the dose selected as the MTD and enables investigation of the working model sensitivity.

Lee and Cheung (2009) proposed a systematic method for calibration of the working model in the CRM based on this indifference interval. Before their method was proposed, the initial guess for the toxicity probability (or the conceptual dose) at each dose level was made by studying the results of comprehensive simulations based on all possible scenarios for the true dose–toxicity relationship before the start of the trial, or was replaced by a guess as indicated by O'Quigley et al. (1990) or Shen and O'Quigley (1996). However, Lee and Cheung (2009) developed a method for determining the initial guess for the toxicity probability at each dose level, given the value of the half-width δ of the indifference interval. When the power model (3.4) is used as the working model, a_k $(k = 1, \ldots, K)$ is obtained as follows, provided the dose corresponding to the MTD based on the initial guess is $d_{k_{0.ig}} \in (k = 1, \ldots, K)$:

$$a_{k+1} = \exp \left(\frac{\log(\Gamma_T + \delta) \log(a_k)}{\log(\Gamma_T - \delta)} \right), \ k = k_{0.ig}, \ldots, K - 1$$

$$a_{k-1} = \exp \left(\frac{\log(\Gamma_T - \delta) \log(a_k)}{\log(\Gamma_T + \delta)} \right) \ k = 2, \ldots, k_{0.ig}.$$

The calibration of δ is based on K scenarios that comprise the dose–toxicity relationships having a plateau shape above and below the lth $(l = 1, \ldots, K)$ dose level, which is the MTD. Specifically, δ is calibrated by performing simulations under these scenarios for candidate values of δ; this step is then followed by selection of a value that maximizes the average across these scenarios of the proportion of trials for which one dose level is selected as the MTD among the total number of trials. Lee and Cheung (2011) proposed a calibration method for the prior distribution in a Bayesian CRM according to the method presented in Lee and Cheung (2009).

3.2.6 Sample Size Determination

The sample size in phase I trials is generally limited to only tens of patients, to speedily move to subsequent phase II trials if there is no concern about toxicity of an agent. The sample size is usually justified or rationalized through simulation with regards to MTD identification or allocation, which is sometimes time-consuming although useful. Methodologies for determining the sample size were proposed by Cheung (2013) and Braun (2018).

3.2.7 For Further Understanding

To quickly acquire a general overview of the CRM, the tutorial paper by Garrett-Mayer (2006) is a useful reference. Furthermore, Ishizuka and Morita (2006) have summarized the practical considerations of the CRM, while O'Quigley (2006a) has summarized the theoretical considerations of the CRM, and O'Quigley (2006b) and O'Quigley and Conaway (2010) have provided comprehensive reviews of designs for the CRM and various extended CRMs. The study by Ishizuka and Ohashi (2001) is also of interest. To deepen one's understanding of the CRM, the book published by Cheung (2011) is useful. In addition, the book written by Crowley and Hoering (2012) discusses some topics relevant to the CRM, related designs, and extended designs. Cheung (2010) has also discussed the similarities and differences between model-based designs and a stochastic approximation design (Robbins and Monro 1951). Finally, the comprehensive review by Thall (2010) focuses more strongly on complex dose-finding designs and should be a useful reference.

3.3 Modified Continual Reassessment Method

3.3.1 Some Issues or Problems with the Original CRM

The original CRM developed by O'Quigley et al. (1990) has been occasionally criticized for the following aspects:

- As an issue that can arise for a Bayesian CRM, the dose recommended for treatment of the first patient in particular is not necessarily safe, especially if the initial guess is incorrect.
- The dose recommended for treatment of patients newly enrolled in the study can be escalated, skipping more than one dose level, compared to the dose administered to the previously enrolled patients. Hence, it is possible that not all dose levels will be investigated, and that a patient could be exposed a dangerous dose.
- To determine the dose to be assigned to the next patient enrolled in the CRM, toxicity evaluation for the previously enrolled patients must be completed. In other words, a certain period of time is required for toxicity evaluation for each patient. Therefore, when a particular patient is within his or her toxicity evaluation period, the toxicity data for that patient naturally does not exist. Thus, it is not possible to determine the dose that should be allocated to the next enrolled patient using the CRM. Under such circumstances, enrollment of a new patient into the trial is suspended. As a result, there are more and longer waiting periods for enrollment to restart, which prolongs the trial.

3.3.2 Dose Skipping, Cohort Size, and Related Issues

Faries (1994) proposed some modifications to the Bayesian CRM in order to allay the aforementioned concerns. The resultant design is called the "modified CRM" or "modified version of the CRM." The modifications are as follows:

1. The next lowest dose level to the level that would be allocated by the CRM is recommended to the next enrolled patient. However, the following exceptions exist:

    a. Dose escalation while skipping at least one dose level is forbidden. In other words, dose escalation involves assignment of the next highest dose level to a level that has already been assigned to an enrolled patient. In particular, the first patient is assigned the lowest dose level from among a set of prespecified dose levels. That is, the dose at the start of the trial is the lowest dose.

    b. If a previously enrolled patient has exhibited a toxic response, patients newly enrolled in the trial are not assigned a dose level higher than that used to treat the patient with the toxic response.

2. As with the 3 + 3 design, the lowest dose level is assigned to not only the first enrolled patient, but also to two other patients, yielding a cohort of three patients.
3. Reference materials for determining the dose allocation include not only data on DLT but also data on mild toxicity.

Korn et al. (1994) focused on the fact that the possibility of treating subjects at a dose level higher than the MTD is greater for the CRM than for the 3 + 3 design, and that the former has a tendency to have a longer trial period, as discussed below. Therefore, in addition to modifications such as those presented in exception 1, Korn et al. (1994) proposed the following modifications to implement the ideas in exception 2 stated above.

1. When a given dose is assigned, it is assigned simultaneously to multiple patients. In other words, the cohort size is greater than one.
2. When a certain number of patients are treated at the dose recommended by the CRM, the MTD is considered to be identified and the trial is suspended earlier.
3. If the minimum dose level cannot be tolerated, an even lower dose level is formally assigned.

Other modifications that have been suggested, but not studied through simulation, include permission of dose escalation for the same patients in subsequent cycles and dose escalation while considering the circumstances in which toxicity less severe than the DLT may arise, as can be seen for subsequently developed accelerated titration designs (Simon et al. 1997) (see Sect. 2.5).

Similar to Faries (1994) and Korn et al. (1994), Goodman et al. (1995) and Møller (1995) also considered some modifications. For example, Goodman et al. (1995) discussed reducing the trial period by enlarging the cohort size without permitting skipping of one or more dose levels. Furthermore, Møller (1995) proposed a modification in which skipping of one or more dose levels is forbidden (in that paper, this approach is called "restriction on the CRM" or "restricted CRM"). Møller (1995) also suggested modifications leading to the development of likelihood-based CRMs (O'Quigley and Shen 1996) (in Møller's work, this approach is called "extension of the CRM" or "extended CRM"). Ahn (1998) also discussed increasing the cohort size and other modifications. During setting of the first stage and post hoc modification, coherence should also be considered as described above for the likelihood-based CRM. That is, if one patient exhibits a toxic response, dose escalation should not be performed for subsequently enrolled patients. For details, see Cheung (2005).

Huang and Chappell (2008) proposed a CRM (LHM-CRM) that allows for assignment of different doses (for example, low, medium, and high doses) to the patients constituting a cohort (for example, a cohort of three patients). Suppose that the low, medium, and high doses assigned to each of the three patients in the $(c + 1)$th cohort for $c = 1, \ldots, C$, i.e., $n = 3C$, are $x_{c+1,L}$, $x_{c+1,M}$, and $x_{c+1,H}$, respectively. In the LMH-CRM, similar to a Bayesian CRM estimation method, the x_{c+1}, l ($l = L, M, H$) assigned to each of the three patients in the $(c + 1)$th cohort are selected to satisfy the following:

$$\left| \psi(x_{c+1,l}, \tilde{\beta}_{c,l}) - \Gamma_{\mathrm{T}} \right| \leq \left| \psi(d_k, \tilde{\beta}_{c,l}) - \Gamma_{\mathrm{T}} \right|; \quad k = 1, \ldots, K, \qquad (3.20)$$

where $\tilde{\beta}_{c,L}$, $\tilde{\beta}_{c,M}$, and $\tilde{\beta}_{c,H}$ are percentiles (for example, 30, 50, and 70%) in the posterior distribution of the MTD, derived from the posterior distribution of β updated using the data acquired until the cth cohort has been completely evaluated for toxicity. However, the patient assigned $x_{c+1,H}$ is exposed to a risk similar to that arising when a dose level is skipped. To avoid this risk, a restriction is imposed to treat patients at doses that do not exceed the highest dose used in the treatment of the cth cohort.

3.3.3 Delayed Outcome and Related Issues

The criticism regarding the delayed outcome described above (see, e.g., O'Quigley et al. 1990, Cheung and Chappell 2000, and Cheung 2005) can be effectively overcome by increasing the cohort size. However, as in the case of a cohort size of 1, complete toxicity data are still required for all patients in a cohort. Thall et al. (1999) proposed two strategies for resolving the issues encountered for the CRM:

1. Based on available data on dose allocation and toxicity outcome, a "look ahead" approach that considers all possible dose assignment and toxicity outcome patterns for future enrolled patients could be implemented. Provided there are no changes to the dose assigned to the next enrolled patient, that dose is assigned to newly enrolled patients without suspending enrollment. If a change is made, enrollment is suspended, but new patients must only wait for enrollment reinitiation for a suitable period of time. If this suitable period of time is exceeded, other treatments are provided separately to the prespecified protocol treatment.
2. When new patients are enrolled, the dose determined by the CRM based only on data from the previously enrolled patients for whom toxicity evaluations are complete is assigned to the new patients as-is (for example, see O'Quigley et al. 1990).

Thall et al. (1999) evaluated the influence of the main performance indices in the CRM, as well as those of the above strategies, on the patient waiting time and the number of patients receiving other treatments not included in the trial protocol. In addition, strategies for enrollment of new patients when there are multiple phase I trials were discussed. Hüsing et al. (2001) also considered the issue of delayed outcomes from a different perspective. Furthermore, Yuan and Yin (2011) proposed a CRM that estimates the toxicity probability using an expectation–maximization (EM) algorithm and considers unevaluated toxicity as missing data.

Piantadosi et al. (1998) considered a CRM in which the working model is a logistic model with two parameters: the slope and the dose associated with a 50% toxicity probability. Hence, they introduced a number of practical modifications to the CRM. Taking the starting dose as the target dose, similar to the approach of O'Quigley et al. (1990), these modifications include a cohort size of at least three and changes during the trial to a dose corresponding to a 90% toxicity probability, taking into account the scenario in which patients experience toxicity at low doses. These modifications can mitigate the risk of treating a patient at a high dose, as noted by Korn et al. (1994) and others. In particular, the latter modification can flexibly expand the upper limit of the dose range to search for a better dose when the toxicity is low. Piantadosi et al. (1998) also introduced some techniques for more practical utilization of these modified CRMs by considering actual examples of clinical trials involving intravenous injection of 9-aminocamptothecin (9-AC) to fresh and recurring cases of malignant glioma. For example, a technique employing a maximum likelihood method to estimate the working model parameters was introduced, in which a prior distribution was empirically constructed through direct incorporation of data on 9-AC dosing and on its associated toxicity from prior studies on the likelihoods of a modified CRM. These data were then combined with data obtained during the trial. In addition, methods for setting the starting dose in modified CRMs utilizing data from prior studies were considered, along with methods for constructing the prior distribution when no such data from prior studies are available.

Potter (2002) noted that situations that are difficult for clinicians to accept may arise in reality, even if the CRM modifications described above are implemented. Specifically, (i) regardless of whether all (or none) of the patients in a given cohort express toxicity, it is possible to assign the same dose level to a newly enrolled cohort and (ii) it is possible to determine the MTD without a single case of toxicity being observed. To avoid these issues, Potter (2002) implemented further modifications to the modified CRM developed by Piantadosi et al. (1998).

Finally, O'Quigley (2009) presented a modified CRM for phase I trials in the field of pediatric oncology, benefitting from the experience of the Pediatric Brain Tumor Consortium. Those researchers discussed methods of addressing the MTD overestimation and parameter estimability problems arising from lack of observed toxicity.

3.3.3.1 Software for Implementation

Software to implement the CRM designs is available as the "dfcrm" R package from https://cran.r-project.org/web/packages/dfcrm/index.html, and as Shiny online applications from http://www.trialdesign.org/. For example, if the target toxicity probability level, data on dose and toxicity, and so on, are provided, we can obtain the dose allocation list, the point estimate and credible interval toxicity probability, and the recommended dose level using the crm function in the dfcrm R package:

```
 1
 2  Create a simple data set
 3  prior <- c(0.05, 0.10, 0.20, 0.35, 0.50, 0.70)
 4  target <- 0.2
 5  level <- c(3, 4, 4, 3, 3, 4, 3, 2, 2, 2)
 6  y <- c(0, 0, 1, 0, 0, 1, 1, 0, 0, 0)
 7  foo <- crm(prior, target, y, level)
 8  ptox <- foo$ptox # updated estimates of toxicity rates
 9  foo
10
11  Today:   Mon Jan 07 19:44:30 2019
12  DATA SUMMARY (CRM)
13  PID       Level    Toxicity        Included
14  1         3        0               1
15  2         4        0               1
16  3         4        1               1
17  4         3        0               1
18  5         3        0               1
19  6         4        1               1
20  7         3        1               1
21  8         2        0               1
22  9         2        0               1
23  10        2        0               1
24
25  Toxicity probability update
26   (with 90 percent probability interval):
27  Level      Prior    n       total.wts
28  1          0.05     0       0
29  2          0.1      3       3
30  3          0.2      4       4
31  4          0.35     3       3
32  5          0.5      0       0
33  6          0.7      0       0
34
35  total.tox          Ptox     LoLmt    UpLmt
36  0                  0.089    0.01     0.283
37  0                  0.155    0.028    0.379
38  1                  0.272    0.082    0.508
39  2                  0.428    0.196    0.643
40  0                  0.571    0.341    0.747
41  0                  0.749    0.574    0.861
42
43  Next recommended dose level: 2
44  Recommendation is based on
45   a target toxicity probability of 0.2
46
```

```
47  Estimation details:
48  Empiric dose-toxicity model: p = dose^{exp(beta)}
49  dose = 0.05 0.1 0.2 0.35 0.5 0.7
50  Normal prior on beta with mean 0 and variance 1.34
51  Posterior mean of beta: -0.212
52  Posterior variance of beta: 0.158
```

This package also allows evaluation of the model sensitivity in the CRM via indifference intervals (see Sect. 3.2.5). Hence, a vector of initial guesses at the toxicity probabilities associated with the doses for a given model sensitivity can be obtained. In addition, simulation results of phase I trials implementing the CRM under a specified dose–toxicity configuration can be generated, the sample size for Bayesian CRM can be calculated, etc.

3.4 Designs Based on Decision Theory or Optimal Design Theory

Whitehead and Brunier (1995) presented a Bayesian decision-theoretic dose-finding design with numerical examples. Rather than focusing on the concept of the MTD in the context of oncological phase I trials, they focused on the dose at which toxicity occurring at a certain frequency can be tolerated in the context of general phase I trials featuring healthy volunteers (who could not benefit from the drug's effects); the dose corresponding to a nontoxic dose outside the context of clinical trials; or the maximum safe dose associated with a tolerable frequency of adverse events.

The design proposed by Whitehead and Brunier (1995) uses a two-parameter logistic model as the working model to configure a parameter prior distribution using pseudo-data; this configuration is based on assumption of an independent beta prior for toxicity probability at each of two dose levels. Therefore, in this sense, the design has a working concept that is fundamentally identical to that of the CRM. One difference from the CRM is that, because the Whitehead and Brunier (1995) design is based on decision theory, dose finding is considered an action, and the decision for that action is based on maximizing the prespecified gain function. For dose x_{j+1} (if K doses $d_1, \ldots, d_K$ are available, $x_{j+1} \in \{d_1, \ldots, d_K\}$) for treatment of the $(j+1)$th patient, in addition to a dose that has already been used to treat all patients up to the jth patient, the gain function $\mathfrak{G}$ is defined by

$$\mathfrak{G}(\beta_0, \beta_1) = \left\{ \mathrm{Var}(x^{\Gamma_\mathrm{T}} | x_{j+1}) \right\}^{-1}, \tag{3.21}$$

where β_0 and β_1 are the parameters of the working model and x^{Γ_T} is the dose corresponding the Γ_T derived from the working model.

When solving Eq. (3.21), each time the $(j+1)$th patient is enrolled in the trial, $\mathrm{Var}(\hat{x}^{\Gamma_\mathrm{T}} | d_k)$ $(k = 1, \ldots, K)$ is calculated using the inverse matrix of the Fisher information matrix accompanying the Taylor approximation of each parameter at the maximum likelihood estimate $\hat{x}^{\Gamma_\mathrm{T}}$ of x^{Γ_T}, because x^{Γ_T} is a function of β_0 and β_1.

However, if this is based on a Bayesian framework, $\mathrm{Var}(\hat{x}^{\Gamma_T}|d_k)$ can be interpreted as the inverse of the variance–covariance matrix from the asymptotic posterior distribution of (β_0, β_1). Thus, it is possible to calculate the value of Eq. (3.21) by substituting the posterior expected values or posterior modes of β_0 and β_1. Consequently, Eq. (3.21) can be regarded as a Bayesian locally c-optimal design from the perspective of optimal design (see Haines et al. 2003).

Based on Eq. (3.21), x^{Γ_T} depends only on the dose used for treatment, not on the binary data on toxicity, and the gain is maximized by the action of assigning a dose to the next enrolled patient that minimizes the dose variance corresponding to Γ_T. Furthermore, Whitehead and Brunier (1995) discussed gain maximization through the action of selecting a dose for the next enrolled patient that minimizes the distance between Γ_T and the estimated toxicity probability, and argued that the CRM is included as a special case in their design. They called the gain obtained in the former case the "variance gain," assuming that the research goal was to improve the dose estimation precision with respect to Γ_T. Similarly, they called the gain acquired in the latter case the "patient gain," regarding the goal as treatment of the patients at the dose corresponding to Γ_T. In particular, the patient gain is suitable for application in the field of oncology, in which it is possible to expose patients to severe toxicity; this approach is equivalent to the dose-finding criteria used in the CRM (Whitehead and Brunier 1995; Whitehead 1997; Whitehead and Williamson 1998).

Whitehead (1997) introduced the same method as discussed above through a retrospective analysis of published data on an oncological trial on quercetin, while providing an overview of the various methods of Bayesian decision theory employed in clinical trials. Whitehead and Williamson (1998) summarized the findings of Whitehead and Brunier (1995) and Whitehead (1997) in a more formal manner, and discussed the elicitation method for prior distributions based on a questionnaire, as well as various prior distributions and gain functions. Furthermore, Zhou and Whitehead (2003) reorganized the findings of the above three published papers, while also discussing suspension criteria based on the ratio between the upper and lower bounds of the confidence interval. Subsequently, Zhou (2005) conducted simulations to investigate the effect of the number of dose levels and cohort sizes on the performance of methods based on the Bayesian decision theory discussed above, and Zhou and Lucini (2005) used simulations to investigate the effect of permitted dose skipping.

To avoid the risk of treating patients with a dangerously high dose, the MTD can be defined as the highest dose with the toxicity probability closest to and not exceeding Γ_T. Thus, Leung and Wang (2002) proposed a decision-theoretic CRM that, based on decision theory, maximizes the expected number of patients (in a trial) treated at the greatest dose that does not exceed Γ_T. If the kth dose level d_k exists and the trials are in the state $\mathfrak{s}_c$ of having transitioned from treatment of the cth cohort ($c = 1, \ldots, C$), let the associated reward be defined as the posterior probability that d_k is the correct MTD. Then, the reward $\mathcal{R}(\mathfrak{s}_c, d_k)$ is given by

$$\mathfrak{R}(\mathfrak{s}_c, d_k) = \begin{cases} \Pr(\psi(d_2, \beta) > \Gamma_T | \mathfrak{s}_c), & k = 1, \\ \Pr(\psi(d_k, \beta) < \Gamma_T, \psi(d_{k+1}, \beta) > \Gamma_T | \mathfrak{s}_c), & k = 2, \ldots, K-1, \\ \Pr(\psi(d_K, \beta) < \Gamma_T | \mathfrak{s}_c), & k = K. \end{cases}$$

$$(3.22)$$

In the decision-theoretic CRM, to maximize the expected number of patients treated at the greatest dose that does not exceed the target toxicity level, the action for the cth cohort is chosen as a continuation ($\mathfrak{C}$) of the same dose as the previous cohort, de-escalation ($\mathfrak{D}$) by one level, and escalation ($\mathfrak{E}$) by one level, so as to maximize the total expected reward as follows:

$$\mathrm{E}(\mathfrak{R}(\mathfrak{s}_1, d_1)) + \sum_{c=2}^{C} \sum_{k=1}^{\min(c,K)} \mathrm{E}(\mathfrak{R}(\mathfrak{s}_c, d_k) \left[I(\mathfrak{C}|\mathfrak{s}_c, d_k) + I(\mathfrak{D}|\mathfrak{s}_c, d_{k+1}) + I(\mathfrak{E}|\mathfrak{s}_c, d_{k-1}) \right]),$$

$$(3.23)$$

where $\mathrm{E}(\cdot)$ represents the expected value of the probability of reaching a particular state and $I(\mathfrak{C}|\mathfrak{s}_c, d_k)$, $I(\mathfrak{D}|\mathfrak{s}_c, d_{k+1})$, and $I(\mathfrak{E}|\mathfrak{s}_c, d_{k-1})$ represent indicator functions in state $\mathfrak{s}_c$. These functions indicate performance of actions $\mathfrak{C}$, $\mathfrak{D}$, or $\mathfrak{E}$ when the dose level is d_k, d_{k+1}, or d_{k-1}, respectively, and $I(\cdot|\cdot, d_0) = I(\cdot|\cdot, d_{K+1}) = 0$.

As discussed above, many dose-finding designs find the MTD or another clinically acceptable dose for the enrolled patient at hand. Thus, these designs emphasize ethics from the individual patient perspective and are, therefore, myopic. However, when considering ethics from the perspective of the patient population, the provision of the MTD or another clinically acceptable dose to future patients cannot be ignored. Bartroff and Lai (2010), Bartroff and Lai (2011) proposed a design that addresses this dilemma.

Furthermore, Haines et al. (2003) presented Bayesian sequential D-optimal and c-optimal designs intended to improve the MTD estimation efficiency. These designs impose constraints that prevent administration of a dangerous dose as indicated by both Babb et al. (1998) and Whitehead et al. (2001). More formally, these designs refine the method of Whitehead and Brunier (1995) using the optimal design theory framework.

3.5 Escalation with Overdose Control Design

Babb et al. (1998) presented the escalation with overdose control (EWOC) design, in which the dose is escalated while protecting patients from receipt of dangerously high doses (or, more specifically, while controlling the chance of subjecting patients to an overdose). Tighiouart et al. (2005) investigated a prior distribution class different from that assumed by Babb et al. (1998) for the EWOC design, and identified the class that can reduce the chances of patient overdose and the risk of toxicity exposure without reducing the MTD estimation performance. Tighiouart and Rogatko (2010) also discussed utilization of large sample characteristics, prior distribution selection, and utilization of covariance in the EWOC design, while introducing examples of their actual application in oncological trials.

The EWOC design assumes a working model with two parameters relating to the MTD and the toxicity probability at the lowest dose (i.e., the trial starting dose), which is obtained by converting the parameters of the tolerance distribution. This design employs a loss function that penalizes overdoses over underdoses, instead of the criteria for dose selection used in the CRM. In this design, for the MTD posterior cumulative distribution function based on obtaining patient data $\mathfrak{D}_j$ for the jth patient, the dose x_j that satisfies the following relation is assigned to patients:

$$\Pr(MTD \leq x_j | \mathfrak{D}_j) = \alpha, \tag{3.24}$$

where α is a prespecified value, say, 0.25. In this manner, the EWOC design differs from the CRM in the prespecification of a working model and gain function, but can still be considered the same with regard to other basic concepts. In fact, a CRM estimating the toxicity probability at the median value of the posterior distribution, while using a two-parameter logistic model as the working model, is equivalent to the EWOC design with $\alpha = 0.5$ (Chu et al. 2009). Chu et al. (2009) presented a hybrid method incorporating the CRM and EWOC designs. Using this method, they succeeded in overcoming an EWOC design problem of MTD underestimation to some extent, by controlling the possibility of treatment at an overdose level. Those researchers also addressed the CRM problem of potential treatment at a dangerously high dose, resulting from mis-specification of both the working model and the prior distribution of its parameters.

3.6 Curve-Free Design

Gasparini and Eisele (2000) presented a curve-free design that assumes a multivariate distribution for $R(d_k)$ at the kth ($k = 1, \ldots, K$) dose level d_k. In this approach, they considered the toxicity monotonicity with regard to the dose rather than appealing to a working model $\psi(x, \beta)$ representing a dose–toxicity response curve and assuming that β follows a certain distribution. In the approach developed by Gasparini and Eisele (2000), clinical investigators first provide an initial guess at $R(d_k)$, as in the CRM. Then, based on parameterization of $R(d_k)$ at certain dose level through the following:

$$\eta_1 = 1 - R(d_1), \quad \eta_i = \frac{1 - R(d_k)}{1 - R(d_{k-1})}; \quad k = 2, \ldots, K, \tag{3.25}$$

it is assumed that η_k ($k = 1, \ldots, K$) independently has a beta distribution. Therefore, $R(d_k) = 1 - \eta_1 \eta_2 \cdots \eta_k$ and the toxicity probability at each dose level is represented as a value associated with the product of the beta distributions. The product of the beta distributions is complex; however, Gasparini and Eisele (2000) obtained its approximation by assuming that this product itself has a beta distribution, in order to acquire the Bayesian estimate for the toxicity probability. Using this estimate, the dose that satisfies the dose selection criteria used in the CRM can be determined. For details of the derivation and specification of the prior distribution, see Gasparini and Eisele (2000). Note these researchers provided corrections to errors in their previous paper in a subsequent work (Gasparini and Eisele 2001). Furthermore, the curve-free design is related to the Bayesian nonparametric design based on the Polya tree process by Muliere and Walker (1997).

However, Cheung (2002) noted the following: In the case that the design accompanying the noninformative prior distribution of Gasparini and Eisele (2000) has a low target toxicity level, a rigidity that holds the doses assigned to patients in the vicinity of suboptimal low doses may occur. Thus, Cheung (2002) provided a solution that utilizes an informative prior distribution through a connection with the CRM. In addition, O'Quigley (2002) argued that curve-free and CRM-based designs are equivalent in that, if certain specifications are given to one design, the other design also features equivalent specifications, despite the fact that the method of discovering such designs is unknown. Here, "equivalent" means that the two specifications have the same operating characteristics.

3.7 Designs Considering Patient Heterogeneity

Phase I trials are generally conducted with a small number of patients and, thus, it is difficult to identify and configure multiple groups by grouping patients by their backgrounds. Even if this were possible, determining separate MTDs for each group may not be particularly meaningful. However, among cancer patients, for example, the particulars of a previous treatment are associated with tolerance to new therapies. Furthermore, it is known that younger acute leukemia patients can tolerate new therapies. In such circumstances, it is meaningful to identify and configure multiple groups by the nature of their previous treatment and age, and to examine the MTD of each group. O'Quigley (1999) presented a two-sample CRM as a methodology for identifying the MTD of each group within a single trial involving two (latent) heterogeneous patient groups. In the two-sample CRM, the one-parameter working model $\psi_1(x, \beta_1)$ used in the conventional CRM is specified for the dose–toxicity relationship in the first group (Group 1). Then, a two-parameter working model $\psi(x, \beta_1, \beta_2)$ is specified for the other group (Group 2). In particular, parameter β_2 has the role of shifting the dose–toxicity response curve of Group 1 and represents the degree of group imbalance. If there are j_1 and j_2 patients in Groups 1 and 2, respectively, yielding a total of $j(= j_1 + j_2)$ patients in both groups, the likelihood based on the data from these patients is

$$\prod_{l=1}^{j_1} \psi_1(x_l, \beta_1)^{y_l} \{1 - \psi_1(x_l, \beta_1)\}^{(1-y_l)} \times \prod_{l=j_1+1}^{j} \psi_2(x_l, \beta_1, \beta_2)^{y_l} \{1 - \psi_2(x_l, \beta_1, \beta_2)\}^{(1-y_l)}.$$

$$(3.26)$$

By maximizing the above likelihood, the maximum likelihood estimate $(\hat{\beta}_{1,j}, \hat{\beta}_{2,j})$ for parameters $(\beta_{1,j}, \beta_{2,j})$ is obtained. (However, note that an initial dose escalation stage is necessary in order to obtain nonuniformity of the presence and absence of toxicity, as in the first stage of the likelihood-based CRM.) Hence, an estimate for the toxicity probability in each group is also obtained, and dose assignment and MTD determination are performed in the same manner as for the ordinary CRM. Two-sample CRMs can be useful if there is a group imbalance and an insufficient number of patients to both specify the CRM working model in each group and to conduct separate trials. O'Quigley and Conaway (2011) indicated that, for the two-sample CRM, it is possible to reduce the working models of O'Quigley et al. (1999) discussed above to a one-parameter working model, by modifying the skeleton. Furthermore, by setting multiple working models (see Sect. 3.9), it is possible to handle patient heterogeneity similarly to the two-sample CRM.

O'Quigley and Paoletti (2003) refined the two-sample CRM to consider the CRM for the case of an ordered relationship between the two samples, in the form of a stronger sensitivity to toxicity in one sample compared to the other. They investigated the influences on the MTD determination for each sample of the choice and mis-specification of the prior distribution for this ordered relationship.

Yuan and Chappell (2004) considered the ordering of multiple groups as well as the monotonicity of the toxicity probability by applying a two-way isotonic regression framework. Then, they proposed a group up-and-down design (see Sect. 2.3), an isotonic design (see Sect. 2.11.3), and an extended CRM allowing for group stratification. Ivanova and Wang (2006) also proposed a nonparametric design based on a bivariate isotonic estimator, which corresponds to the two-sample CRM or an ordered two-sample CRM.

Morita et al. (2017) evaluated a design based on the Bayesian hierarchical model, a generalization of the CRM, which can take into account situations where the dose–toxicity relationships are exchangeable between subgroups. Chapple and Thall (2018) proposed a design, called Sub-TITE, for phase I trials with a time-to-toxicity outcome and two or more subgroups, which allows subgroup-specific dose decision while combining subgroups with similar dose–toxicity relationships. Software to implement the Sub-TITE designs is available as the "SubTite" R package from https://cran.r-project.org/web/packages/SubTite/index.html.

3.8 Designs Considering Pharmacokinetic or Patient Background Information

Use of information regarding patient pharmacokinetics can aid understanding of the relationship between dose and toxicity (Christian and Korn 1994). Piantadosi and Liu (1996) assumed a logistic model as the CRM working model and suggested incorporating the area under the curve (AUC) of the serum drug concentration as a covariate. The corresponding working model is given by

$$\psi(x, b_c, \beta_1, \beta_2) = \frac{1}{1 + \exp(b_c - \beta_1 x - \beta_2 \Delta AUC),} \tag{3.27}$$

where b_c gives the odds ratio of the baseline toxicity probability and is fixed to a constant, although $b_c > 0$. Here, β_1 and β_2 are parameters related to the administered dose and observed AUC, respectively, and $\beta_1 > 0$ and $\beta_2 > 0$. These can be estimated in a Bayesian framework. In addition, x is the dose assigned to the patients; $\Delta AUC = AUC - x/\kappa$, where AUC is the actually observed AUC for treatment of patients at dose x. The term x/κ is derived by assuming a two-compartment model for the *in vivo* pharmacokinetics, where κ is the rate constant when the drug is lost from the blood compartment. From Eq. (3.27), the toxicity probability increases with the dose administered to the patients or with the observed AUC. As a result, the risk of treatment at a dangerously high dose can be avoided by considering the AUC. In addition, instead of the AUC, pharmacokinetic information on the maximum serum drug concentration or the time to reach that concentration can be used. However, one difficulty in implementing this design is the need to measure pharmacokinetic information in real time.

For the case of phase I trials involving healthy volunteers and a treatment agent for attention deficit hyperactivity disorder, Whitehead et al. (2007) used a linear mixed-effects model to describe the relationship between the AUC as a pharmacokinetic indicator and each of the toxicity and pharmacodynamic responses (here defined as the degree of pulse rate increase from the baseline), so as to predict the action mechanism of the drug. Those researchers argued for a Bayesian design based on this model. Using this design, it is possible to identify a dose that yields a pharmacologically desirable treatment while controlling the predictive probabilities of the AUC and toxicity exceeding respective thresholds. On this topic, Bailey (2009a) presented a dose escalation design for the case of a large intercohort difference in a first-in-man trial with healthy volunteers as subjects (see also discussions by O'Quigley (2009) and Bailey (2009b) on the Bailey (2009a) study).

It is also possible to incorporate patient background information or pretreatment observations as covariates into the working model (Wijesinha and Piantadosi 1995; Christian and Korn 1994). For example, Legedza and Ibrahim (2001) presented a Bayesian estimation method for the patient-specific MTD and the population-averaged MTD from this perspective. In this method, an informative prior distribution is specified using the likelihood based on patient background information as well as data on the dose and presence or absence of toxicity for individual patients obtained from previous trials (Whitehead 2002). Hence, a methodology for inputting the informative prior into the CRM was developed while controlling the precision using the fixed value of a power parameter. Babb and Rogatko (2001) presented a design for adjusting the dose used to treat patients. The approach presented in that study derived the dose–toxicity relationship for each patient by incorporating the covariate of the anti-Staphylococcus aureus exotoxin antibody concentrations for the patients' pretreatment into the working model of an EWOC design (see also, Rogatko et al. 2008). This design can be considered to be an extended version of the EWOC design that considers personalized therapy.

3.9 Designs with Multiple-Candidate Dose–Toxicity Models

Shen and O'Quigley (1996) indicated that, for large sample sizes, the CRM is robust against mis-specification of the working model and that the doses recommended by the CRM converge to the true MTD. However, this type of asymptotic behavior cannot be considered to be particularly appropriate for phase I trials conducted with several tens of patients at most. Consequently, the initial guess at the toxicity probability at each dose level affects the CRM operating characteristics. Yin and Yuan (2009a) developed a Bayesian model averaging CRM (BMA-CRM), which allows for multiple working models (more specifically, those researchers investigated the initial guess for the toxicity probability in a power model (Eq. (3.4)). Through averaging of these working models, the BMA-CRM is robust against an incorrect initial guess at the toxicity probability (see Pan and Yuan (2017) for the specification of multiple working models).

Let us consider M working models $\mathfrak{M}_1, \ldots, \mathfrak{M}_M$:

$$\mathfrak{M}_m : \ \psi_m(d_k, \beta) = a_{m,k}^{\exp(\beta_m)}; \ m = 1, \ldots, M, \ k = 1, \ldots, K, \tag{3.28}$$

where $a_{m,k}$ is the initial guess for the toxicity probability at dose level k in the mth working model, with $0 < a_{m,1} < \ldots < a_{m,K} < 1$. Further, β_m is a parameter in the mth working model, where $-\infty < \beta_m < \infty$. If the prior probability of the mth working model is $\Pr(\mathfrak{M}_m)$, then, given data $\mathfrak{D}_j$ up to the jth patient, the posterior probability $\Pr(\mathfrak{M}_m | \mathfrak{D}_j)$ of the mth working model is given by

$$\Pr(\mathfrak{M}_m | \mathfrak{D}_j) = \frac{\bar{\mathfrak{L}}_{m,j}(a_m)\Pr(\mathfrak{M}_m)}{\sum_{m=1}^{M} \bar{\mathfrak{L}}_{m,j}(a_m)\Pr(\mathfrak{M}_m)}, \tag{3.29}$$

where $\bar{\mathfrak{L}}_{m,j}(\beta_m)$ is the marginal likelihood for the mth working model. This marginal likelihood is given by

$$\bar{\mathfrak{L}}_{m,j}(\beta) = \int_{-\infty}^{\infty} \mathfrak{L}_{m,j}(\beta_m) g(\beta_m | \mathfrak{M}_m) d\beta_m, \tag{3.30}$$

where $\mathfrak{L}_{m,j}(\beta_m) = \prod_{l=1}^{j} \{\psi_m(x_l, \beta_m)\}^{y_l} \{1 - \psi_m(x_l, \beta_m)\}^{(1-y_l)}$, and $g(\beta_m | \mathfrak{M}_m)$ is the prior distribution of parameter β_m given the mth working model M_m. In the BMA-CRM, using the posterior probability of the working model, the toxicity probability at dose level k ($k = 1, \ldots, K$) is estimated from

$$\tilde{R}(d_k) = \sum_{m=1}^{M} \tilde{R}_m(d_k)\Pr(\mathfrak{M}_m | \mathfrak{D}_j), \tag{3.31}$$

where $\tilde{R}_m(d_k)$ is the estimated toxicity probability in the Bayesian CRM for the mth working model. As can be understood from Eq. (3.31), the toxicity probability is estimated by using the posterior probabilities of the models to weight the estimates for the toxicity probability in the CRM based on each working model. Daimon et al. (2011) presented the CRM based on the model selection. In addition, O'Quigley and Conaway (2011) discussed comprehensive handling of the partial ordering for multiple treatment schedules, patient heterogeneity, and drug combinations (see Sect. 3.14) by utilizing an extended CRM based on Eq. (3.29). Furthermore, Yuan and Yin (2011) proposed an extended CRM that estimates the dose–toxicity relationship by handling the toxicity outcome that has not been observed as missing data. Then, an expectation–maximization algorithm as well as model averaging is applied.

Software for implementing the BMA-CRM designs is available as a stand-alone graphical user interface-based Windows desktop program from https://biostatistics.mdanderson.org/SoftwareDownload/SingleSoftware.aspx?Software_Id=81, and as Shiny online applications from http://www.trialdesign.org/.

3.10 Designs for Late-Onset Toxicity Outcome

Most designs for phase I trials including the CRM determine the dose for a newly enrolled patient or cohort by completely observing the presence or absence of toxicity in each patient. In trials evaluating the late-onset toxicity of radiotherapy and preventive agents, long-term follow-up is needed until observations regarding the presence or absence of toxicity is complete; thus, such trials have long duration.

Cheung and Chappell (2000) considered the time-to-toxicity and developed a time-to-event CRM (TITE-CRM) as an extended CRM. In this approach, doses can be assigned to newly enrolled patients or cohorts without waiting for complete observations of the presence or absence of toxicity. In the TITE-CRM, instead of the one-parameter model $\psi(x, \beta)$ used in the CRM, the CRM is extended by considering a weighted working model $\psi(x, w, \beta)$, which increases monotonically with weight w. The log-likelihood function in the TITE-CRM can be obtained by substituting $\psi(x, w, \beta)$ for $\psi(x, \beta)$ (see Sect. 3.2). One simple potential form of $\psi(x, w, \beta)$ is to associate w with $\psi(x, \beta)$ as a proportionality coefficient satisfying $0 \leq w \leq 1$: $\psi(x, w, \beta) = w\psi(x, \beta)$. By considering the time until toxicity is observed in each patient, w is given as a function of the time until toxicity observation, denoted by T, and of the time until toxicity is actually observed, denoted by t as follows:

$$w(t; T) = \frac{t}{T}. \tag{3.32}$$

This function is expected to work well in a number of circumstances, but can be considered to be excessively simplified. Therefore, Cheung and Chappell (2000) also provided a function for addressing late-onset toxicity and dose-dependent and parameter-dependent functions.

However, although it is possible to anticipate whether the toxicity being evaluated is late or early onset to some extent and according to the treatment type, there are also cases when this aspect is dose dependent. As a result, it is difficult to discern whether the toxicity in question is late or early onset and to select an appropriate corresponding function during trial planning. Furthermore, it is even more difficult to discern late- or early-onset toxicity because only a subset of treated patients experience toxicity. Therefore, it may ultimately be difficult to select and use the weighted function described above ahead of time. Braun (2006) was motivated by this issue and generalized the TITE-CRM, in which a data-adaptively weighted function that does not require a prior specification of late or early onset is used. This is achieved by assuming that the time until toxicity onset has a beta distribution and, also, by allowing one of the parameters to depend on the dose.

The TITE-CRM has another problem. As indicated by Cheung and Chappell (2000), while waiting to collect toxicity information from treated patients, the patient accumulation is not suspended. Therefore, if the patient accumulation speed is high and the toxicity is late onset, future patients could be exposed to dangerously high doses. To solve this problem, Bekele et al. (2008) presented a predicted risk of toxicity (PRT) method that uses a predictive probability to quantify the PRT at a dose to be administered to a future patient or the dose at the next level. If this predictive probability has an unacceptable value, the trials are temporarily suspended and toxicity information is obtained; otherwise, enrollment is restarted. This PRT method finds a point of compromise between the CRM problem that a complete toxicity evaluation is required, with registration being forbidden until this information is obtained, and the TITE-CRM problem that a complete toxicity evaluation is not required and enrollment with incomplete toxicity information is permitted. Thus, the PRT method indicates the length of time for which patient enrollment should be suspended during toxicity information acquisition. However, Polley (2011) subsequently noted that the PRT method is mathematically complex and requires specialized computer programs and data collection infrastructure; thus, Polley (2011) presented a simpler, modified method.

Braun et al. (2003) presented a modified TITE-CRM designed to find the maximum tolerated cumulative dose (MTCD) (instead of the MTD) of the recombinant human keratinocyte growth factor; the aim was to mitigate the chemotherapy-induced damage on the mucosa-lined tissue of the lower gastrointestinal tract in allogeneic bone marrow transplantation trials. Mauguen et al. (2011) developed a time-to-event EWOC design in the same manner as the CRM expansion to the TITE-CRM. In addition, Zhao et al. (2011) showed that, in the field of pediatric oncology, the TITE-CRM has superior performance to the rolling-6 design (Skolnik et al. 2008).

Liu et al. (2013) proposed the data augmentation continual reassessment method (DA-CRM), in which unobserved toxicities are treated as missing data, and the Bayesian data augmentation approach is used to sample both the missing data and model parameters from their posterior full conditional distributions.

Software to implement the TITE-CRM design is available in the "dfcrm" R package from https://cran.r-project.org/web/packages/dfcrm/index.html. Further, software to implement the DA-CRM design together with the CRM and BMA-CRM designs is available as a stand-alone graphical user interface-based Windows desktop program from https://biostatistics.mdanderson.org/softwaredownload/SingleSoft ware.aspx?Software_Id=132.

3.11 Designs for Ordinal or Continuous Toxicity Outcomes

In oncological trials, toxicity is categorized by grades ordered by severity in accordance with the National Cancer Institute Common Terminology Criteria for Adverse Events (NCI-CTCAE). However, in oncological phase I trials that aim to determine the MTD, these grades are dichotomized depending on whether they constitute DLT. For example, grade-4 fatigue is considered DLT, but grades 0–3 are not. In addition, this type of dichotomization works well in the case of relatively mild toxicity that resolves if the treatment is suspended, such as neutropenia. Both grade-3 and -4 neutropenia may be considered DLT, but the difference between these two grades is not generally considered important. However, this is unlikely to be the case for severe and irreversible forms of toxicity such as nephrotoxicity, hepatotoxicity, and neurotoxicity. For example, grade-4 acute kidney failure requires dialysis and, thus, constitutes a far more dangerous form of toxicity than grade-3. Depending on the type of toxicity, if there are fears that a grade-2 case will progress to grades 3 and 4, this naturally occupies the attention of clinical investigators. Consequently, some clinical investigators may decide to escalate or de-escalate the dose of the agent of interest in an oncological phase I trial, considering the grade information instead of dichotomized data only. In addition, utilization of grade information may yield improved performance of the employed dose-finding design (Paoletti et al. 2004).

Various designs considering the toxicity grade have been presented. For example, Wang et al. (2000) presented a modified CRM that modifies the likelihood to reflect the relative severity of toxicity using grades 3 and 4 and that weights Γ_T.

Bekele and Thall (2004) discussed the advantages of utilizing information on the toxicity types and individual grades in trials for determining the preoperative MTD of gemcitabine alongside external irradiation for soft-tissue sarcoma patients. They proposed consideration of the severity weight on a numerical scale with values that are 0 or higher, depending on the toxicity type and grade. They also suggested defining their sum as the total toxicity burden (TTB), and performing dose-finding based on this TTB. In that approach, a Bayesian multivariate ordinal probit model is used to simultaneously address the ordinal response of the toxicity, the latent variables that specify the correlation structure between toxicities, and the random variables for the severity weight.

Yuan et al. (2007) proposed the quasi-CRM, in which the severity weight of the toxicity is used to convert the grades into a numeric score; these scores are then incorporated into a CRM using a quasi-Bernoulli likelihood. In the quasi-CRM, the concept of an algorithm with a threshold for the number of patients experiencing toxicity in the cohort (similar to the 3 + 3 design) is utilized, and an equivalent toxicity (ET) score is introduced to measure the relative severity of the toxicity grades having different thresholds. Suppose that the cutoff grade for identifying the toxicity as DLT in a given trial is grade-3, and that the target toxicity level is 33%. This cutoff grade is given an ET score of 1. All toxicity patterns that can occur in a cohort of three subjects (for example, a combination of grade 0 for the first subject, grade-2 for the second subject, and grade-4 for the third subject) are listed, and escalation, de-escalation, or maintenance of the dose for each of these combinations is decided by clinical investigators. Hence, the ET score is established for grades other than grade-3. For example, (i) toxicity at grade-1 is of no concern, (ii) toxicity at grade-2 in two patients is equivalent to toxicity at grade 3 in one patient, and (iii) toxicity at grade-2 in one patient and at grade-4 in one patient is equivalent to toxicity at grade-3 in two patients. In this case, as grade-3 is given a score of 1, grades 2 and 4 are assigned scores of 0.5 and 1.5, respectively.

Let Y^{ET} denote the ET score. The normalized ET score Y^{nET} is expressed as

$$Y^{nET} = Y^{ET}/Y^{ET}_{max}, \tag{3.33}$$

where $Y^{ET}_{max} < \infty$ is the ET score for the most severe grade. Consequently, $Y^{nET} \in [0, 1]$. In addition, similar to specification of a working model for the dose–toxicity relationship in the CRM, the relationship between the dose and the normalized ET score for dose x is

$$R^{nET}(x) = E(Y^{nET}|x) = \psi^{nET}(x, \beta),$$

where $R^{nET}(x)$ is the true normalized ET score for dose x, $\psi^{nET}(x, \beta)$ is the working model for the relationship between the dose and the normalized ET score, and β is a parameter. Compared to the binary toxicity Y in the CRM, Y^{nET} can be considered to divide the interval of $[0, 1]$, thereby reconsidering a binary event as a fractional event. Here, by replacing Y with Y^{nET} and $\psi(x, \beta)$ with $\psi^{nET}(x, \beta)$ in the Bernoulli likelihood, a quasi-Bernoulli likelihood is obtained. The quasi-CRM finds the dose at which the estimated normalized ET score is closest to the target-normalized ET score based on this pseudo-likelihood. By modifying the score function in Eq. (3.33), the quasi-CRM can also be applied to toxicity expressed not as an ordinal category, but rather as a continuous quantity. In addition, it seems that the ET score itself can be applied to situations using the $3 + 3$ design (Yuan et al. 2007). The ET score has also been discussed by Chen et al. (2010), including its application in an isotonic method.

Bekele et al. (2010) proposed a dose-finding design that considers the toxicity grade when there are multiple risk groups due to differences in toxicity sensitivity among the subjects; this is achieved by using an average toxicity score similar to that employed in the approach developed by Bekele and Thall (2004). In addition, van Meter et al. (2011) presented a dose-finding design that considers the NCI-CTCAE grade information by replacing the working model in the CRM with a proportional odds model.

Ivanova (2006) considered an algorithm-based dose-finding design for use when the toxicity is evaluated as ordinal categorical data. Furthermore, Ivanova and Kim (2009) specified a function requiring only monotonicity in the relationship between dose and toxicity, for data obtained in binary, ordinal, or continuous form, and proposed a unified approach toward dose finding with respect to toxicity obtained in the form of these data. Ivanova and Murphy (2009) also provided an application example of these designs to an NGX267 trial for Alzheimer's disease treatment in healthy male volunteers.

Lee et al. (2011) proposed an extended CRM that can be applied when a single toxicity occurrence is observed as binary, ordinal categorical, or continuous data, and also when multiple toxicity results are given in terms of the TTB, by imposing multiple toxicity constraints. Finally, Iasonos et al. (2011) discussed use of toxicity information at grades lower than the DLT in a two-stage CRM.

3.12 Designs for Determination of Maximum Tolerated Schedule

In the case of late-onset toxicity, a long-term observation period is required; thus, long trial periods tend to occur. The TITE-CRM is effective for determining the maximum tolerated dose under such circumstances. However, this method considers toxicity that is evaluated based on the administration of a single dose or a single course of an agent, similar to the conventional CRM. Thus, this design cannot be used to study toxicity evaluated based on administration of multiple doses or multiple courses of the target drug. Braun et al. (2005) discussed this problem in relation to allogeneic bone marrow translation trials; hence, they presented a method for finding the maximum tolerated schedule (MTS) as an evaluation index based on observations of long-term toxicity response for an agent across multiple doses or multiple courses. Use of the MTS is in contrast to use of the MTD, which is an evaluation index based on short-term observations of toxicity for drugs administered once. Here, the term "schedule" refers to the total number of drug administration cycles, and the toxicity risk exposure resulting from this schedule is given as the sum of the hazards of toxicity in each cycle constituting the schedule. The individual hazard functions are represented by triangular functions with three parameters. Braun et al. (2003) previously presented a separate method for MTS determination. In this method, each schedule is considered to be a single dose, and the TITE-CRM is applied with accommodation of dose escalation within individuals. However, as discussed by Braun et al. (2005), as schedule extension within individuals is permitted, it is unclear which dose contributes to the late-onset toxicity.

A limitation of the design by Braun et al. (2005) is that the dose within each administered course must be fixed at the same value for all patients. If this fixed dose is poor, the resultant MTS becomes far from optimal. In oncological phase I trials, the treatment protocol generally consists of multiple courses. Changes to dosing, such as de-escalation or skipping, can be made depending on those courses and in accordance with the dosing criteria or patient condition. Thus, their design is a novel method in the sense that it can determine the MTS, but cannot be considered suitable for such circumstances. To solve these problems, Braun et al. (2007) proposed a design that finds the maximum tolerated dose and schedule by permitting adjustment of not only the courses of administration, but also the doses, on a per-patient basis. This approach reflects the actual treatment protocol employed in the trials. This method is a generalization of Braun et al. (2005).

3.13 Review of Design Performance Comparisons

O'Quigley and Chevret (1991), Korn et al. (1994), Goodman et al. (1995), Ahn (1998), Iasonos et al. (2008), and others have compared the performance of various designs, including the $3+3$ (see Sect. 2.2) and CRM (see Sects. 3.2 and 3.3) designs. In the above works, excluding that by Korn et al. (1994), the CRM was concluded to have favorable performance compared to the $3+3$ design. However, Korn et al. (1994) argued that the CRM has longer trial periods than the $3+3$ design and is unsafe; thus, they recommended use of the $3+3$ design. Subsequently, O'Quigley (1999) noted a number of defects in the investigation performed by Korn et al. (1994) and, after re-examination, argued that the conclusion of those authors was erroneous (see also, Iasonos and O'Quigley 2011). However, Korn et al. (1999) offered a rebuttal.

Gerke and Siedentop (2008a) used simulations to evaluate the performance of various designs for dose finding in oncological phase I trials focusing on toxicity evaluation alone. The considered methods were the $3+3$ design, likelihood-based CRM, and Bayesian ADEPT (this is a software package, although the naming gives the erroneous impression that it is a statistical method, as cautioned by Shu and O'Quigley 2008). Gerke and Siedentop (2008a) argued that, although the simulation results showed identical trends to a number of findings reported in the above-mentioned design comparison studies, there is no support for the superiority of the likelihood-based CRM over the $3+3$ design as regards MTD identification. Instead, those authors argued that Bayesian ADEPT is superior to the $3+3$ design. Nevertheless, Shu and O'Quigley (2008) offered a strong rebuttal, stating that the CRM-related investigation and simulations conducted by Gerke and Siedentop (2008a) were insufficient to yield results supporting use of Bayesian ADEPT. Gerke and Siedentop (2008b) later replied in the form of a rebuttal.

Skolnik et al. (2008) proposed the rolling-6 design and compared its performance with that of the $3+3$ design and the CRM. While noting problems concerning adjustment of the administered dose based on body surface area in the field of pediatric oncology, Onar-Thomas and Xiong (2010) later conducted a more thorough performance comparison that included the CRM; those researchers considered incorporation of the body surface area into the designs proposed by Skolnik et al. (2008). Hence, no major differences between the rolling-6 design, $3+3$ design, and CRM were found in terms of toxicity frequency. It was also concluded that the rolling-6 design is quicker than the $3+3$ design as regards MTD estimation, but slower than the CRM. It was also found that the rolling-6 design and CRM have shorter trial periods than the $3 + 3$ design, and that the CRM has a shorter trial period than the rolling-6 method when the patient recruitment is particularly fast. Thus, although advantages of the rolling-6 design are found relative to the $3 + 3$ design, there seems to be no apparent advantages to its use over the CRM.

3.14 Designs for Drug Combinations

Cancer therapy includes surgical therapy, chemotherapy, radiotherapy, immunotherapy, etc., but curative treatment of cancer using just one of these therapies is difficult. Consequently, rather than a treatment involving one therapy or one drug, use of multidisciplinary treatments that combine various therapies or combination therapies that combine multiple treatments is common in practice. For example, chemotherapy treatment is performed by combining multiple drugs having different properties. Naturally, the type and specifics (the dose or schedule in the case of treatment involving drugs) of the treatments employed in multidisciplinary or combination therapies must be such that the patients are provided with an optimal combination with tolerable toxicity (and, depending on the circumstances, in the manner that yields the greatest therapeutic effect) (see, e.g., Hamberg and Verweij 2009). One advantage of such combination therapies is that a synergistic therapeutic effect can be obtained while suppressing toxicity when multiple drugs are employed; this is because one treatment amplifies the intensity or sensitivity of another treatment. Other advantages include the fact that different sensitivities can be expected from various drugs without cross-tolerance, and that the treatment intensity can be increased if toxicity overlapping can be avoided (Korn and Simon 1993).

Examples of combination therapy designs involving two drugs (Drugs 1 and 2) that find dose combinations yielding a toxicity probability close to Γ_T are given in the form of an annotated bibliography below.

Simon and Korn (1990, 1991) proposed a method for finding combinations of anticancer drugs and their doses from the perspective of dose intensity. Those researchers also argued for the use of a tolerable-dose diagram in the trial protocol for combination therapy (Korn and Simon 1993). A possible, simple design is to fix the Drug 1 dose and escalate the Drug 2 dose. Then, when the tolerable dose of Drug 2 is identified, the Drug 1 dose can be escalated (Korn and Simon 1993). However, this method does not necessarily identify the optimal combination among all possible combinations. Furthermore, considerable effort is required for trial implementation in cases where there are many candidate dose levels for each drug.

Kramar et al. (1999) investigated the possibility of applying the CRM to the design of a trial of combination therapy involving docetaxel and irinotecan. In that study, simulations and a retrospective analysis using the CRM were performed based on data from phase I trials evaluating the safety of combination therapy involving these two drugs, which were conducted using the $3 + 3$ design. The modifications made in this case were (1) to identify a dose combination for the two drugs with an order constraint that satisfies the assumption of monotonicity of the toxicity probability, as required by the CRM and (2) to select the dose levels to reflect this combination (utilizing the benefit of the CRM that the dose levels merely act as a label) so that the CRM could be applied. However, this design can only be used to study dose combinations of two drugs having an order constraint, to allow application of the CRM. Note that Su (2010) introduced a simple method that includes modifications to a two-stage CRM.

Thall et al. (2003) proposed a dose-finding trial design for combination therapy involving gemcitabine and cyclophosphamide. In that approach, to indicate the toxicity probability for the dose combinations, a six-parameter model that features the standardized doses for each drug and their interactions as explanatory variables is assumed. A two-stage search is conducted over two-dimensional coordinates for which the standardized doses for each drug are taken as axes. In the first stage, a search for a dose combination of both drugs is performed on a straight line with simultaneous increases or decreases of both drug doses. In the second stage, in addition to the straight-line search, a further search is performed on a contour line along which the toxicity probability becomes equal to Γ_T.

Wang and Ivanova (2005) proposed a design that finds the maximum tolerated combination (MTC) with respect to toxicity, while identifying the MTD for one of the two drugs corresponding to each dose of the other drug. Let $d_{1,1}, \ldots, d_{1,K_1}$ denote K_1 available doses for Drug 1, and $d_{2,1}, \ldots, d_{2,K_2}$ denote K_2 available doses for Drug 2. In the Wang and Ivanova (2005) method, the following working model is assumed:

$$\psi(d_{1,k_1}, d_{2,k_2}, \beta_1, \beta_2, \beta_3) = 1 - (1 - a_{1,k_1})^{\beta_1} (1 - a_{2,k_2})^{\beta_2 + \beta_3 \log(1 - a_{1,k_1})};$$
$$k_1 = 1, \ldots, K_1, \ k_2 = 1, \ldots, K_2,$$
$$(3.34)$$

where $0 < a_{1,1} < \ldots < a_{1,K_1} < 1; 0 < a_{2,1} < \ldots < a_{2,K_2} < 1$; and β_1, β_2, and β_3 are the parameters. For the working model for Eq. (3.34) to satisfy the assumption of monotonicity for the toxicity probability, $\beta_1 > 0$, $\beta_2 > 0$, and $\beta_3 > 0$. However, $\beta_3 = 0$ corresponds to the case that the doses of the two drugs have no interaction effect. The parameters and toxicity probability are estimated as in a Bayesian CRM.

Yuan and Yin (2008) presented a dose-finding design that sequentially conducts subtrials instead of investigating all dose combinations of the two drugs. For K_1 dose levels $d_{1,1} < \ldots < d_{1,K1}$ of Drug 1 and K_2 dose levels $d_{2,1} < \ldots < d_{2,K2}$ of Drug 2, $d_{1,k_1} d_{2,k_2}$ represents the Drug 1 dose corresponding to dose level k_1 and the Drug 2 dose corresponding to dose level k_2. If $k_1 \leq k_1'$ and $k_2 \leq k_2'$, the toxicity of $d_{1,k_1} d_{2,k_2}$ is assumed to be lower or identical to that of $d_{1,k_1'} d_{2,k_2'}$. When all combinations of the two drug doses are studied, the simplest procedure is to search for the MTD of Drug 2 based on fixing of the Drug 1 dose at each dose level. This is equivalent to performing K_1 dose-finding trials and determining the MTD of Drug 2 in each of them. Trials involving one-dimensional dose finding of one drug based on fixing of the dose of the other can be regarded as subtrials within a two-dimensional dose-finding trial for two drugs. Let $d_{1,k_1} d_{2,s \to t}$ denote the subtrials used to find the corresponding doses from dose level s to t for Drug 2. Then, the two-dimensional dose-finding trial for investigating all dose combinations for the two drugs can be denoted by $\{d_{1,1}d_{2,1\to K_2}, \ldots, d_{1,K_1}d_{2,1\to K_2}\}$.

The dose-finding algorithm is described as follows, with the CRM being used in each subtrial:

Step 1 K_1 subtrials $\{d_{1,1}d_{2,1\to K_2}, \ldots, d_{1,K_1}d_{2,1\to K_2}\}$ are divided into subtrial groups of size three, for example, $\{d_{1,1}\,d_{2,1\to K_2},\, d_{1,2}\,d_{2,1\to K_2},\, d_{1,3}\,d_{2,1\to K_2}\}$, $\{d_{1,4}d_{2,1\to K_2}, d_{1,5}d_{2,1\to K_2}, d_{1,6}d_{2,1\to K_2}\}$, etc. Each subtrial is called the "low-," "medium-," and "high-dose subtrial" in accordance with the Drug 1 dose level in the subtrials for the different groups (for example, in the first subtrial group, these correspond to $d_{1,1}d_{2,1\to K_2}, d_{1,2}d_{B,1\to K_2}$, and $d_{1,3}d_{2,1\to K_2}$, respectively).

Step 2 Conduct the subtrials for the first subtrial group as follows:

(2a) Conduct the medium-dose subtrial $d_{1,2}d_{2,1\to K_2}$ and identify the MTD.

(2b) Once this MTD is identified as $d_{1,2}d_{2,k_{2,2}^*}$, simultaneously conduct the low-$d_{1,1}d_{2,k_{2,2}^*\to K_2}$ and high-dose $d_{1,3}d_{2,1\to k_{2,2}^*}$ subtrials, and identify the MTD for each subtrial.

(2c) If all combinations in $d_{1,2}d_{2,1\to k_2}$ have excessive toxicity and the MTD cannot be identified, conduct the low-dose subtrial $d_{1,1}d_{1\to K_2}$ to search for the MTD. Subsequently, this subtrial in the first subtrial group is terminated.

Step 3 If the MTD of $d_{1,3}d_{2,1\to k_{2,2}^*}$ is identified as $d_{1,3}d_{2,k_{2,3}^*}$, use the same method as in Step 2 to conduct the subtrials in the second subtrial group, while appropriately setting the dose level boundaries for Drug 2. That is, start with $d_{1,5}d_{2,1\to k_{2,3}^*}$. If the MTD is identified as $d_{1,5}d_{2,k_{2,5}^*}$, simultaneously conduct the low-dose $d_{1,4}d_{2,k_{2,5}^*\to k_{2,3}^*}$ and high-dose $d_{1,6}d_{2,1\to k_{2,5}^*}$ subtrials to determine their respective MTDs.

This design can narrow the MTD search range for one drug, while reducing the sample size, if the patient accumulation speed is not particularly high. In addition, because the dose of one drug is determined relative to a fixed dose for the other drug, multiple dose combination candidates are obtained.

Yin and Yuan (2009b) noted that, although each of the two drugs has different toxicities, the specific drug that causes a particular toxicity cannot necessarily be identified; thus, overlap between drugs is possible depending on the type of toxicity (in other words, if toxicity is observed, it is difficult to identify the source drug). Those researchers presented a design that assumes a latent 2×2 contingency table for this possibility. Furthermore, by using a Gumbel model (Murtaugh and Fisher 1990) for the toxicity probability pattern of the two drugs represented by that contingency table, this approach estimates the toxicity probabilities of the combination therapy resulting from combination of various doses of the two drugs. The working model for the toxicity probability for each drug is a power model (3.4). The MTD combination for the two drugs in the combination therapy is selected as the dose combination at which the estimated toxicity probability is closest to Γ_T, as in the CRM. Furthermore, Yin and Yuan (2009c) presented a dose–toxicity relationship for each drug using a power model (Eq. (3.4)) as the working model, and used various copula models (see Clayton 1978, Hougaard 1986, and Genest and Rivest 1993) to link the toxicity probabilities of each drug to the toxicity probabilities of the combination therapy. Hence, they performed dose finding among the dose combinations for the two drugs.

Bailey et al. (2009) conducted a case study of combination therapy with two drugs. By assuming the model proposed by Neuenschwander et al. (2008) for the dose–toxicity relationship of imatinib and incorporating a covariate on the amount of administered nilotinib, a pair of MTDs for the respective drugs was identified for combination therapy using both.

Braun and Wang (2010) proposed a method for finding the MTC by assuming a beta distribution for the toxicity probabilities of dose combinations of the two drugs. In this approach, a Bayesian hierarchical model is adopted after logarithmic transformation of the parameters that have the doses of the two drugs as explanatory variables; the hyperparameters are assumed to have a multivariate normal distribution. Wheeler et al. (2019) proposed the product of independent beta probabilities escalation design for combination therapy with two drugs, focusing on censored time-to-toxicity outcomes.

Although it is difficult to find the full ordering of the toxicity probabilities with respect to all dose combinations in combination therapy involving two drugs, Conaway et al. (2004) noted that it is possible to find the known partial ordering within the full ordering. Those researchers discussed a nonparametric design that finds dose combinations for two drugs by exploiting information on this partial ordering. Fan et al. (2009) presented an algorithm for expanding the search range for candidate combinations according to Conaway et al. (2004), and presented two- and three-stage designs that further consider the low-grade toxicity information. Changes to the dose combinations are performed using a $3 + 3$ design and its variant in the form of a $2 + 1 + 3$ design, and the toxicity probability is estimated based on an isotonic estimator. Note that Braun and Alonzo (2011) presented a more generalized $A + B + C$ design.

Wages et al. (2011a, b) proposed Bayesian and likelihood CRMs exploiting information on the partial ordering in Conaway et al. (2004). In this design, potential full orderings are configured from known partial orderings for the combination of the two drugs, which are regarded as working models. Then, the optimal working model (full ordering) is selected from the obtained patient data, and dose combinations are found based on that working model.

3.15 Related Topics

3.15.1 Retrospective Analysis

Ishizuka and Ohashi (2001) first presented an example of prospective CRM application to an actual phase I trial. Until those results were produced, the advantages of the CRM were mostly discussed based on simulations. In some cases, to evaluate the operating characteristics, retrospective analysis of data acquired in trials implemented under a design different from the CRM (e.g., the $3 + 3$ design) was performed using the CRM. Because the dose allocation and toxicity evaluation were conducted prospectively and sequentially, this kind of retrospective analysis was merely a reference for elucidating the CRM operating characteristics. On the other hand, implementation of this kind of retrospective analysis likely raised questions on the CRM behavior and the dose finally determined as the MTD. Such questions can also arise under the following circumstances:

- when switching to the CRM from a different design while trials are underway, such that the obtained data so far are used in the CRM;
- when incorporating data obtained from other trials or cohorts in the CRM; and
- when data obtained from trials conducted using the CRM are re-analyzed using CRMs based on various working models to evaluate their robustness.

Dose allocation and MTD determination are performed sequentially and prospectively in accordance with the design adopted in the trial planning. Thus, it is not possible to retrospectively return to the data after trial completion (even hypothetically) based on a design different from that adopted in planning, e.g., in order to directly retrace the trial of interest. Motivated by this problem, O'Quigley (2005) presented a methodology for estimating the MTD through retrospective application of the CRM (rCRM). He used a weighted average across dose levels to reconsider the derivative of the log-likelihood function in the CRM (Eqs. (3.17) and (3.18)).

After obtaining data up to the jth patient, let $\hat{\omega}_j(d_k)$ denote the relative frequency of patients treated at the kth dose level d_k among j patients, for $k = 1, \ldots, K$. By replacing n with j and x_j with d_k in $U_j(\beta)$ in Eq. (3.18), it is possible to rewrite this expression as

$$
U_j(\beta) = \sum_{k=1}^{K} I\left(\left(\sum_{l=1}^{j} I(x_l = d_k)\right) \neq 0\right) \hat{\omega}_j(d_k)
$$
$$
\times \left[\frac{\sum_{l=1}^{j} y_l I(x_l = d_k)}{\sum_{l=1}^{j} I(x_l = d_k)} \frac{\psi'}{\psi} \{d_k, \beta\} \right.
$$
$$
\left. + \left\{ 1 - \frac{\sum_{l=1}^{j} y_l I(x_l = d_k)}{\sum_{l=1}^{j} I(x_l = d_k)} \right\} \frac{-\psi'}{1 - \psi} \{d_k, \beta\} \right], \qquad (3.35)
$$

where $I(\cdot)$ is an indicator function having a value of 1 if the conditions in parentheses are satisfied; otherwise, it takes a value of 0. Furthermore, $\hat{\omega}_j(d_k)$ acts as a weight when the average across the dose levels is taken. If the data are obtained under a CRM design, with increasing j, $\hat{\omega}_j(d_k) \to 0$ and $\hat{\omega}_j(d_0) \to 1$ at all d_k satisfying $d_k \neq d_0$, where d_0 is the true MTD (Shen and O'Quigley 1996). Of course, the $\hat{\omega}_j(d_k)$ distribution differs for small and large sample sizes, but these properties are suitably satisfied (Onar et al. 2009). However, if the trials are actually conducted under a different design, this approach is not necessarily applicable. Thus, O'Quigley considered adjusting $\hat{\omega}_j(d_k)$ with a more appropriate weight and solving an estimation equation, i.e., Eq. (3.35), with the right-hand side set to zero in order to estimate the parameter in the working model. Note that, in this case, the appropriate weight is obtained by conducting simulations such that the true toxicity probability at each dose level is $\hat{R}(d_k) = \sum_{l=1}^{j} y_l I(x_l = d_k) / \sum_{l=1}^{j} I(x_l = d_k)$.

O'Quigley and Zohar (2010) evaluated the robustness of the rCRM for the third circumstance listed above. In addition, Zohar et al. (2011) presented a methodology for utilizing the rCRM as a tool for meta-analysis combining the results (MTDs) of multiple oncological phase I trials.

However, some problems that arise during application of the rCRM are as follows:

- In the CRM, the toxicity probability is assumed to increase monotonically with dose, but the actually obtained $\hat{R}(d_k)$ is not necessarily monotonic. Thus, there are cases in which no solutions of the weighted estimation equation based on Eq. (3.35) exist. Smoothing using isotonic regression is also possible, but $\hat{R}(d_k)$ is forced to be uniform at some dose levels; thus, a performance improvement cannot be expected.
- The CRM is subject to some modifications when applied, as seen in Sect. 3.3; thus, it is necessary to consider a weight that considers those modifications.

Iasonos and O'Quigley (2011) noted these issues and proposed a constrained maximum likelihood estimation that controls the increments in toxicity probability between neighboring dose levels as an alternative to the rCRM.

3.15.2 Optimal Design

The operating characteristics of dose-finding designs are evaluated using simulations of hypothetical trials under various scenarios, while considering the true relationship between the dose and toxicity probability that can be encountered in practice. The emphasis is on safe determination of the MTD or the optimal dose to be administered to the patients, and on trial design that allows early termination when appropriate. Therefore, the indices concerning the design operating characteristics commonly evaluated in the simulations are the following: (i) the proportion of trials in which each dose level is selected as the MTD across all trials, (ii) the average patient proportion treated at each dose level out of the prespecified sample size of each trial across all trials, (iii) the average patient proportion across all trials that experiences toxicity out of the prespecified sample size in each trial, (iv) the mean squared error between the toxicity probability at the estimated MTD and target toxicity probability level, and so on. By using these indices, the operating characteristics of different designs can be compared and their superiority or inferiority can be discussed.

O'Quigley et al. (2002) proposed use of a nonparametric optimal design based on contrasting incomplete and complete information as a technique for comparing operating characteristics among designs. Here, incomplete information is that for which the information state is missing. In other words, for K available dose levels $d_1, \ldots, d_K$ and based on the assumption that the toxicity increases monotonically with dose, if toxicity occurs in a patient at d_k ($k \leq K$), it will always occur at d_l ($k \leq l \leq K$). However, information is lacking as to whether toxicity will occur at dose levels lower than d_k. On the other hand, if toxicity does not occur at d_k ($1 \leq k$), it will never occur at d_l ($1 \leq l \leq k$). However, information is lacking as to whether it will occur at dose levels higher than d_k. Meanwhile, the complete information indicates the state in which all information is available. In other words, this refers to the state in which toxicity information has been obtained for all dose levels for each patient. Of course, this type of complete information is not actually available, but it can be obtained in simulations. Specifically, given the threshold v_j (generated from random numbers with a uniform distribution) of the toxicity probability that can be tolerated for a dose for the jth patient, the occurrence of toxicity $Y_j(d_k)$ at each dose level d_k is given by

$$Y_j(d_k) = \begin{cases} 0, & v_j > R(d_k) \\ 1, & v_j \leq R(d_k) \end{cases}, \tag{3.36}$$

and the true toxicity probability at the kth dose level is estimated by

$$\widehat{R}(d_k) = \frac{1}{n} \sum_{j=1}^{n} Y_j(d_k). \tag{3.37}$$

Note that, because $R(d_1) \leq \ldots \leq R(d_k)$, $\widehat{R}(d_1) \leq \ldots \leq \widehat{R}(d_k)$. Then, the MTD estimated by the optimal design based on complete information is identified as the dose that minimizes $|\widehat{R}(d_k) - \Gamma_T|$; this is similar to the criteria for dose selection in the CRM (see Eq. (3.2)). As a result, it is also possible to evaluate the operating characteristics of the optimal design through simulations using the indices described above.

With complete information, it is possible to obtain empirical estimates for the true toxicity probability without using a parametric model; thus, this approach is nonparametric in this sense. In addition, the estimate is unbiased and its variance attains the Cramér–Rao lower bound. In this sense, this design using complete information is "optimal." The data obtained in practice indeed constitute incomplete information; thus, the nonparametric optimal design is merely a conceptual tool that cannot be applied to actual trials. However, when applying a design for MTD identification, or when investigating potential improvement of multiple-candidate designs, this nonparametric optimal design is useful in that it acts as a benchmark.

As a tool for evaluating the operating characteristics other than the optimal design, O'Quigley et al. (2002) and Paoletti et al. (2004) introduced a measure from the perspective of efficiency, and presented a graphical display of the cumulative distribution for the difference between the toxicity probability at the estimated MTD and Γ_T.

References

Ahn, C.: An evaluation of phase I cancer clinical trial designs. Stat. Med. **17**(14), 1537–1549 (1998)

Asakawa, T., Ishizuka, N., Hamada, C.: A continual reassessment method that adaptively changes the prior distribution according to the initial cohort observation. Jpn. J. Clin. Pharmacol. Ther. **43**(1), 21–28 (2012)

Babb, J.S., Rogatko, A.: Patient specific dosing in a cancer phase I clinical trial. Stat. Med. **20**(14), 2079–2090 (2001)

Babb, J., Rogatko, A., Zacks, S.: Cancer phase I clinical trials: efficient dose escalation with overdose control. Stat. Med. **17**(10), 1103–1120 (1998)

Bailey, R.A.: Designs for dose-escalation trials with quantitative responses. Stat. Med. **28**(30), 3721–3738 (2009a)

Bailey, R.A.: Authors' rejoinder to Commentaries on 'Designs for dose-escalation trials with quantitative responses'. Stat. Med. **28**(30), 3759–3760 (2009b)

Bailey, S., Neuenschwander, B., Laird, G., Branson, M.: A Bayesian case study in oncology phase I combination dose-finding using logistic regression with covariates. J. Biopharm. Stat. **19**(3), 469–484 (2009)

Bartroff, J., Lai, T.L.: Approximate dynamic programming and its applications to the design of phase I cancer trials. Stat. Sci. **25**(2), 245–257 (2010)

Bartroff, J., Lai, T.L.: Incorporating individual and collective ethics into phase I cancer trial designs. Biometrics **67**(2), 596–603 (2011)

Bekele, B.N., Ji, Y., Shen, Y., Thall, P.F.: Monitoring late-onset toxicities in phase I trials using predicted risks. Biostatistics **9**(3), 442–457 (2008)

Bekele, B.N., Li, Y., Ji, Y.: Risk-group-specific dose finding based on an average toxicity score. Biometrics **66**(2), 541–548 (2010)

Bekele, B.N., Thall, P.F.: Dose-finding based on multiple toxicities in a soft tissue sarcoma trial. J. Am. Stat. Assoc. **99**(465), 26–35 (2004)

Bensadon, M., O'Quigley, J.: Integral evaluation for continual reassessment method. Comput. Programs. Biomed. **42**(4), 271–273 (1994)

Braun, T.M.: Generalizing the TITE-CRM to adapt for early- and late-onset toxicities. Stat. Med. **25**(12), 2071–2083 (2006)

Braun, T.M.: Motivating sample sizes in adaptive phase 1 trials via Bayesian posterior credible intervals. Biometrics. **74**(3), 1065–1071 (2018)

Braun, T.M., Alonzo, T.A.: Beyond the 3+3 method: expanded algorithms for dose-escalation in phase I oncology trials of two agents. Clin. Trials **8**(3), 247–259 (2011)

Braun, T.M., Levine, J.E., Ferrara, J.L.M.: Determining a maximum tolerated cumulative dose: dose reassignment within the TITE-CRM. Control. Clin. Trials **24**(6), 669–681 (2003)

Braun, T.M., Thall, P.F., Nguyen, H., de Lima, M.: Simultaneously optimizing dose and schedule of a new cytotoxic agent. Clin. Trials **4**(2), 113–124 (2007)

Braun, T.M., Wang, S.: A hierarchical Bayesian design for phase I trials of novel combinations of cancer therapeutic agents. Biometrics **66**(3), 805–812 (2010)

Braun, T.M., Yuan, Z., Thall, P.F.: Determining a maximum-tolerated schedule of a cytotoxic agent. Biometrics **61**(2), 335–343 (2005)

Chapple, A.G., Thall, P.F.: Subgroup- specific dose finding in phase I clinical trials based on time to toxicity allowing adaptive subgroup combination. Pharm. Stat. **17**(6), 734–749 (2018)

Chen, Z., Krailo, M.D., Azen, S.P., Tighiouart, M.: A novel toxicity scoring system treating toxicity response as a quasi-continuous variable in phase I clinical trials. Contemp. Clin. Trials **31**(5), 473–482 (2010)

Cheung, Y.K.: On the use of nonparametric curves in phase I trials with low toxicity tolerance. Biometrics **58**(1), 237–240 (2002)

Cheung, Y.K.: Coherence principles in dose-finding studies. Biometrika **92**(4), 863–873 (2005)

Cheung, Y.K.: Stochastic approximation and modern model-based designs for dose-finding clinical trials. Stat. Sci. **25**(2), 191–201 (2010)

Cheung, Y.K.: Dose Finding by the Continual Reassessment Method. Chapman and Hall/CRC Press, Boca Raton, FL (2011)

Cheung, Y.: Sample size formulae for the Bayesian continual reassessment method. Clin. Trials **10**(6), 852–861 (2013)

Cheung, Y.K., Chappell, R.: Sequential designs for phase I clinical trials with late-onset toxicities. Biometrics **56**(4), 1177–1182 (2000)

Cheung, Y.K., Chappell, R.: A simple technique to evaluate model sensitivity in the continual reassessment method. Biometrics **58**(3), 671–674 (2002)

Chevret, S.: The continual reassessment method in cancer phase I clinical trials: a simulation study. Stat. Med. **12**(12), 1093–1108 (1993)

Christian, M.C., Korn, E.L.: The limited precision of phase I trial. J. Nat. Cancer Inst. **86**(2), 1662–1663 (1994)

Chu, P.-L., Lin, Y., Shih, W.J.: Unifying CRM and EWOC designs for phase I cancer clinical trials. J. Stat. Plan. Inference **139**(3), 1146–1163 (2009)

Clayton, D.G.: A model for association in bivariate life tables and its application in epidemiological studies of familial tendency in chronic disease incidence. Biometrika **65**(1), 141–152 (1978)

Collins, J.M., Zaharko, D.S., Dedrick, R.L., Chabner, B.A.: Potential roles for preclinical pharmacology in phase I clinical trials. Cancer Treat. Rep. **70**(1), 73–80 (1986)

Conaway, M.R., Dunbar, S., Peddada, S.D.: Designs for single- or multiple-agent phase I trials. Biometrics **60**(3), 661–669 (2004)

Crowley, J., Hoering, A.: Handbook of Statistics in Clinical Oncology, 3rd edn. Chapman and Hall/CRC Press, Boca Raton, FL (2012)

Daimon, T., Zohar, S., O'Quigley, J.: Posterior maximization and averaging for Bayesian working model choice in the continual reassessment method. Stat. Med. **30**(13), 1563–1573 (2011)

Edler, L., Burkholder, I.: Chapter 1. Overview of phase I trials. In: Crowley, J., Ankerst, D.P. (eds.) Handbook of Statistics in Clinical Oncology, 2nd edn., pp. 1–29. Chapman and Hall/CRC Press, Boca Raton, FL (2006)

Fan, K., Venookb, A.P., Lu, Y.: Design issues in dose-finding phase I trials for combinations of two agents. J. Biopharm. Stat. **19**(3), 509–523 (2009)

Faries, D.: Practical modifications of the continual reassessment method for phase I cancer clinical trials. J. Biopharm. Stat. **4**(2), 147–164 (1994)

Garrett-Mayer, E.: The continual reassessment method for dose-finding studies: a tutorial. Clin. Trials **3**(1), 57–71 (2006)

Gasparini, M., Eisele, J.: A curve-free method for phase I clinical trials. Biometrics **56**(2), 609–615 (2000)

Gasparini, M., Eisele, J.: Correction to "A curve-free method for phase I clinical trials" by M. Gasparini and J. Eisele (2000). Biometrics **57**(2), 659–660 (2001)

Gatsonis, C., Greenhouse, J.B.: Bayesian methods for phase I clinical trials. Stat. Med. **11**(10), 1377–1389 (1992)

Genest, C., Rivest, L.-P.: Statistical inference procedures for bivariate Archimedean copulas. J. Am. Stat. Assoc. **88**(423), 1034–1043 (1993)

Gerke, O., Siedentop, H.: Optimal phase I dose-escalation trial designs in oncology: a simulation study. Stat. Med. **27**(26), 5329–5344 (2008a)

Gerke, O., Siedentop, H.: Authors' rejoinder to 'Dose-escalation designs in oncology: ADEPT and the CRM'. Stat. Med. **27**(26), 5354–5355 (2008b)

Goodman, S.N., Zahurak, M.L., Piantadosi, S.: Some practical improvements in the continual reassessment method for phase I studies. Stat. Med. **14**(11), 1149–1161 (1995)

Haines, L.M., Perevozskaya, I., Rosenberger, W.F.: Bayesian decision procedures for dose determining experiments. Biometrics **59**(3), 591–600 (2003)

Hamberg, P., Verweij, J.: Phase I drug combination trial design: walking the tightrope. J. Clin. Oncol. **27**(27), 4441–4443 (2009)

Hougaard, P.: A class of multivariate failure time distributions. Biometrika **73**(3), 671–678 (1986)

Huang, B., Chappell, R.: Three-dose-cohort designs in cancer phase I trials. Stat. Med. **27**(12), 2070–2093 (2008)

Hüsing, J., Sauerwein, W., Hideghéty, K., Jöckel, K.-H.: A scheme for a dose-escalation study when the event is lagged. Stat. Med. **20**(22), 3323–3334 (2001)

Iasonos, A., O'Quigley, J.: Continual reassessment and related designs in dose-finding studies. Stat. Med. **30**(17), 2057–2061 (2011)

Iasonos, A., Ostrovnaya, I.: Estimating the dose-toxicity curve in completed phase I studies. Stat. Med. **30**(17), 2117–2129 (2011)

Iasonos, A., Zohar, S., O'Quigley, J.: Incorporating lower grade toxicity information into dose finding designs. Clin. Trials **8**(4), 370–379 (2011)

Iasonos, A., Wilton, A.S., Riedel, E.R., Seshan, V.E., Spriggs, D.R.: A comprehensive comparison of the continual reassessment method to the standard $3 + 3$ dose escalation scheme in phase I dose-finding studies. Clin. Trials **5**(5), 465–477 (2008)

Ishizuka, N., Morita, S.: Practical implementation of the continual reassessment method. In: Crowley, J., Ankerst, D.P. (eds.) Handbook of Statistics in Clinical Oncology, 2nd edn., pp. 31–58. Chapman and Hall/CRC Press, Boca Raton, FL (2006)

Ishizuka, N., Ohashi, Y.: The continual reassessment method and its applications: a Bayesian methodology for phase I cancer clinical trials. Stat. Med. **20**(17–18), 2661–2681 (2001)

Ivanova, A.: Escalation, group and $A + B$ designs for dose-finding trials. Stat. Med. **25**(21), 3668–3678 (2006)

Ivanova, A., Kim, S.H.: Dose finding for continuous and ordinal outcomes with a monotone objective function: a unified approach. Biometrics **65**(1), 307–315 (2009)

Ivanova, A., Murphy, M.: An adaptive first in man dose-escalation study of NGX267: statistical, clinical, and operational considerations. J. Biopharm. Stat. **19**(2), 247–255 (2009)

Ivanova, A., Wang, K.: Bivariate isotonic design for dose-finding with ordered groups. Stat. Med. **25**(12), 2018–2026 (2006)

Korn, E.L., Midthune, D., Chen, T.T., Rubinstein, L.V., Christian, M.C., Simon, R.M.: A comparison of two phase I trial designs. Stat. Med. **13**(8), 1799–1806 (1994)

Korn, E.L., Midthune, D., Chen, T.T., Rubinstein, L.V., Christian, M.C., Simon, R.M.: Commentary. Stat. Med. **18**(20), 2691–2692 (1999)

Korn, E.L., Simon, R.: Using the tolerable-dose diagram in the design of phase I combination chemotherapy trials. J. Clin. Oncol. **11**(4), 794–801 (1993)

Kramar, A., Lebecq, A., Candalh, E.: Continual reassessment methods in phase I trials of the combination of two drugs in oncology. Stat. Med. **18**(14), 1849–1864 (1999)

Lee, S.M., Cheung, Y.K.: Model calibration in the continual reassessment method. Clin. Trials **6**(3), 227–238 (2009)

Lee, S.M., Cheung, Y.K.: Calibration of prior variance in the Bayesian continual reassessment method. Stat. Med. **30**(17), 2081–2089 (2011)

Lee, S.M., Cheng, B., Cheung, Y.K.: Continual reassessment method with multiple toxicity constraints. Biostatistics **12**(2), 386–398 (2011)

Legedza, A.T.R., Ibrahim, J.G.: Heterogeneity in phase I clinical trials: prior elicitation and computing using the continual reassessment method. Stat. Med. **20**(6), 867–882 (2001)

Leung, D., Wang, Y.-G.: An extension of the continual reassessment method using decision theory. Stat. Med. **21**(1), 51–63 (2002)

Liu, S., Yin, G., Yuan, Y.: Bayesian data augmentation dose finding with continual reassessment method and delayed toxicity. Ann. Appl. Stat. **7**(4), 2138–2156 (2013)

Mauguen, A., Le Deley, M.C., Zohar, S.: Dose-finding approach for dose escalation with overdose control considering incomplete observations. Stat. Med. **30**(13), 1584–1594 (2011)

Morita, S.: Application of the continual reassessment method to a phase I dose-finding trial in Japanese patients: East meets West. Stat. Med. **30**(17), 2090–2097 (2011)

Morita, S., Thall, P.F., Müller, P.: Determining the effective sample size of a parametric prior. Biometrics **64**(2), 595–602 (2008)

Morita, S., Thall, P.F., Takeda, K.: A simulation study of methods for selecting subgroup-specific doses in phase 1 trials. Pharm. Stat. **16**(2), 143–156 (2017)

Møller, S.: An extension of the continual reassessment method using a preliminary up and down design in a dose-finding study in cancer patients in order to investigate a greater number of dose levels. Stat. Med. **14**(9), 911–922 (1995)

Muliere, P., Walker, S.: A Bayesian nonparametric approach to determining a maximum tolerated dose. J. Stat. Plan. Inference **61**(2), 339–353 (1997)

Murphy, J.R., Hall, D.L.: A logistic dose-ranging method for phase I clinical investigations trials. J. Biopharm. Stat. **7**(4), 635–647 (1997)

Murtaugh, P.A., Fisher, L.D.: Bivariate binary models of efficacy and toxicity in dose-ranging trials. Commun. Stat. Theory Methods **19**(6), 2003–2020 (1990)

Natarajan, L., O'Quigley, J.: Interval estimates of the probability of toxicity at the maximum tolerated dose for small samples. Stat. Med. **22**(11), 1829–1836 (2003)

Neuenschwander, B., Branson, M., Gsponer, T.: Critical aspects of the Bayesian approach to phase I cancer trials. Stat. Med. **27**(13), 2420–2439 (2008)

Onar A., Kocak, M., Boyett, J.M.: Continual reassessment method vs. traditional empirically-based design: modifications motivated by phase I trials in pediatric oncology by the Pediatric Brain Tumor Consortium. J. Biopharm. Stat. **19**(3), 437–455 (2009)

Onar-Thomas, A., Xiong, Z.: A simulation-based comparison of the traditional method, rolling-6 design and a frequentist version of the continual reassessment method with special attention to trial duration in pediatric phase I oncology trials. Contemp. Clin. Trials **31**(3), 259–270 (2010)

O'Quigley, J.: Estimating the probability of toxicity at the recommended dose following a phase I clinical trial in cancer. Biometrics **48**(3), 853–862 (1992)

O'Quigley, J.: Another look at two phase I clinical trial designs. Stat. Med. **18**(20), 2683–2690 (1999)

O'Quigley, J.: Curve-free and model-based continual reassessment method designs. Biometrics **58**(1), 245–249 (2002)

O'Quigley, J.: Retrospective analysis of sequential dose-finding designs. Biometrics **61**(3), 749–756 (2005)

O'Quigley, J.: Theoretical study of the continual reassessment method. J. Stat. Plan. Inference **136**(6), 1765–1780 (2006a)

O'Quigley, J.: Chapter 2. Phase I and phase I/II dose finding algorithms using continual reassessment method. In: Crowley, J., Ankerst D.P. (eds.) Handbook of Statistics in Clinical Oncology, 2nd edn., pp. 31–58. Chapman and Hall/CRC Press, Boca Raton, FL (2006b)

O'Quigley, J.: Commentary on 'Designs for dose-escalation trials with quantitative responses'. Stat. Med. **28**(30), 3745–3750; discussion 3759–3760 (2009)

O'Quigley, J., Chevret, S.: Methods for dose finding studies in cancer clinical trials: a review. Stat. Med. **10**(11), 1647–1664 (1991)

O'Quigley, J., Conaway, M.: Continual reassessment method and related dose-finding designs. Stat. Sci. **25**(2), 202–216 (2010)

O'Quigley, J., Conaway, M.: Extended model-based designs for more complex dose-finding studies. Stat. Med. **30**(17), 2062–2069 (2011)

O'Quigley, J., Paoletti, X.: Continual reassessment method for ordered groups. Biometrics **59**(2), 430–440 (2003)

O'Quigley, J., Paoletti, X., Maccario, J.: Non-parametric optimal design in dose finding studies. Biostatistics **3**(1), 51–56 (2002)

O'Quigley, J., Pepe, M., Fisher, L.: Continual reassessment method: a practical design for phase 1 clinical trials in cancer. Biometrics **46**(1), 33–48 (1990)

O'Quigley, J., Shen, L.Z.: Continual reassessment method: a likelihood approach. Biometrics **52**(2), 673–684 (1996)

O'Quigley, J., Shen, L.Z., Gamst, A.: Two-sample continual reassessment method. J. Biopharm. Stat. **9**(1), 17–44 (1999)

O'Quigley, J., Zohar, S.: Retrospective robustness of the continual reassessment method. J. Biopharm. Stat. **20**(5), 1013–1025 (2010)

Pan, H., Yuan, Y.: A default method to specify skeletons for Bayesian model averaging continual reassessment method for phase I clinical trials. Stat. Med. **36**(2), 266–279 (2017)

Paoletti, X., O'Quigley, J., Maccario, J.: Design efficiency in dose finding studies. Comput. Stat. Data Anal. **45**(2), 197–214 (2004)

Paoletti, X., Baron, B., Schöffski, P., Fumoleau, P., Lacombe, D., Marreaud, S., Sylvester, R.: Using the continual reassessment method: Lessons learned from an EORTC phase I dose finding study. Eur. J. Cancer **42**(10), 1362–1368 (2006)

Paoletti, X., Kramar, A.: A comparison of model choices for the continual reassessment method in phase I cancer trials. Stat. Med. **28**(24), 3012–3028 (2009)

Piantadosi, S., Liu, G.: Improved designs for dose escalation studies using pharmacokinetic measurements. Stat. Med. **15**(15), 1605–1618 (1996)

Piantadosi, S., Fisher, J.D., Grossman, S.: Practical implementation of a modified continual reassessment method for dose-finding trials. Cancer Chemother. Pharmacol. **41**(6), 429–436 (1998)

Polley, M.-Y.C.: Practical modifications to the time-to-event continual reassessment method for phase I cancer trials with fast patient accrual and late-onset toxicities. Stat. Med. **30**(17), 2130–2143 (2011)

Potter, D.M.: Adaptive dose finding for phase I clinical trials of drug used for chemotherapy of cancer. Stat. Med. **21**(13), 1805–1823 (2002)

Resche-Rigon, M., Zohar, S., Chevret, S.: Adaptive designs for dose-finding in non-cancer phase II trials: influence of early unexpected outcomes. Clin. Trials **5**(6), 595–606 (2008)

Robbins, H., Monro, S.: A stochastic approximation method. Ann. Math. Stat. **22**(3), 400–407 (1951)

Rogatko, A., Ghosh, P., Vidakovic, B., Tighiouart, M.: Patient-specific dose adjustment in the cancer clinical trial setting. Pharmaceut. Med. **22**(6), 345–350 (2008)

Shen, L.Z., O'Quigley, J.: Consistency of continual reassessment method under model misspecification. Biometrika **83**(2), 395–405 (1996)

Shu, J., O'Quigley, J.: Commentary: dose-escalation designs in oncology: ADEPT and the CRM. Stat. Med. **27**(26), 5345–5353 (2008)

Silvapulle, M.J.: On the existence of maximum likelihood estimators for the binomial response models. J. Royal Stat. Soc. Series B **43**(3), 310–313 (1981)

Simon, R., Korn, E.L.: Selecting drug combinations based on total equivalent dose (dose intensity). J. Nat. Cancer Inst. **82**(18), 1469–1476 (1990)

Simon, R., Korn, E.L.: Selecting combinations of chemotherapeutic drugs to maximize dose intensity. J. Biopharm. Stat. **1**(2), 247–259 (1991)

Simon, R.M., Freidlin, B., Rubinstein, L., Arbuck, S.G., Collins, J., Christian, M.C.: Accelerated titration designs for phase I clinical trials in oncology. J. Nat. Cancer Inst. **89**(15), 1138–1147 (1997)

Skolnik, J.M., Barrett, J.S., Jayaraman, B., Patel, D., Adamson, P.C.: Shortening the timeline of pediatric phase I trials: the rolling six design. J. Clin. Oncol. **26**(2), 190–195 (2008)

Storer, B.E.: Design and analysis of phase I clinical trials. Biometrics **45**(3), 925–937 (1989)

Su, Z.: A two-stage algorithm for designing phase I cancer clinical trials for two new molecular entities. Contemp. Clin. Trials **31**(1), 105–107 (2010)

Takeda, K., Morita, S.: Bayesian dose-finding phase I trial design incorporating historical data from a preceding trial. Pharm. Stat. **17**(4), 372–382 (2018)

Thall, P.F.: Bayesian models and decision algorithms for complex early phase clinical trials. Stat Sci. **25**(2), 227–244 (2010)

Thall, P.F., Lee, J.J., Tseng, C.-H., Estey, E.H.: Accrual strategies for phase I trials with delayed patient outcome. Stat. Med. **18**(10), 1155–1169 (1999)

Thall, P.F., Millikan, R.E., Mueller, P., Lee, S.-J.: Dose-finding with two agents in phase I oncology trials. Biometrics **59**(3), 487–496 (2003)

Tighiouart, M., Rogatko, A., Babb, J.S.: Flexible Bayesian methods for cancer phase I clinical trials. Dose escalation with overdose control. Stat. Med. **24**(14), 2183–2196 (2005)

Tighiouart, M., Rogatko, A.: Dose finding with escalation with overdose control (EWOC) in cancer clinical trials. Stat. Sci. **25**(2), 217–226 (2010)

van Meter, E.M., Garrett-Meyer, E., Bandyopadhyay, D.: Proportional odds model for dose-finding clinical trial designs with ordinal toxicity grading. Stat. Med. **30**(17), 2070–2080 (2011)

Wages, N.A., Conaway, M.R., O'Quigley, J.: Continual reassessment method for partial ordering. Biometrics **67**(4), 1555–1563 (2011a)

Wages, N.A., Conaway, M.R., O'Quigley, J.: Dose-finding design for multi-drug combinations. Clin. Trials **8**(4), 380–389 (2011b)

Wang, C., Chen, T., Tyan, I.: Designs for phase I cancer clinical trials with differentiation of graded toxicity. Commun. Stat. Theory Methods **29**(5–6), 975–987 (2000)

Wang, O., Faries, D.E.: A two-stage dose selection strategy in phase I trials with wide dose ranges. J. Biopharm. Stat. **10**(3), 319–333 (2000)

Wang, K., Ivanova, A.: Two-dimensional dose finding in discrete dose space. Biometrics **61**(1), 217–222 (2005)

Wheeler, G.M., Sweeting, M.J., Mander, A.P.: A Bayesian model free–approach to combination therapy phase I trials using censored time- to- toxicity data. J. R. Stat. Soc. Ser. C Appl. Stat. **68**(2), 309–329 (2019)

Whitehead, J.: Bayesian decision procedures with application to dose-finding studies. Int. J. Pharm. Med. **11**, 201–208 (1997)

Whitehead, J.: Letter to the editor: "Heterogeneity in phase I clinical trials: prior elicitation and computation using the continual reassessment method" by Legedza, A., Ibrahim, J.G. (2001), Stat. Med. **20**(6), 867–882. Stat. Med. **21**(8), 1172 (2002)

Whitehead, J., Brunier, H.: Bayesian decision procedures for dose determining experiments. Stat. Med. **14**(9–10), 885–893 (1995)

Whitehead, J., Williamson, D.: Bayesian decision procedures based on logistic regression models for dose-finding studies. J. Biopharm. Stat. **8**(3), 445–467 (1998)

Whitehead, J., Zhou, Y., Hampson, L., Ledent, E., Pereira, A.: A Bayesian approach for dose-escalation in a phase I clinical trial incorporating pharmacodynamic endpoints. J. Biopharm. Stat. **17**(6), 1117–1129 (2007)

Whitehead, J., Zhou, Y., Patterson, S., Webber, D., Francis, S.: Easy-to-implement Bayesian methods for dose-escalation studies in healthy volunteers. Biostatistics **2**(1), 47–61 (2001)

Wijesinha, M.C., Piantadosi, S.: Dose-response models with covariates. Biometrics **51**(3), 977–987 (1995)

Yin, G., Yuan, Y.: Bayesian model averaging continual reassessment method in phase I clinical trials. J. Am. Stat. Assoc. **104**(487), 954–968 (2009a)

Yin, G., Yuan, Y.: A latent contingency table approach to dose-finding for combinations of two agents. Biometrics **65**(3), 866–875 (2009b)

Yin, G., Yuan, Y. Bayesian dose finding for drug combinations by copula regression. J. Roy. Stat. Soc. Ser. C Appl. Stat. **58**(2), 211–224 (2009c)

Yuan, Z., Chappell, R.: Isotonic designs for phase I cancer clinical trials with multiple risk groups. Clin. Trials **1**(6), 499–508 (2004)

Yuan, Z., Chappell, R., Bailey, H.: The continual reassessment method for multiple toxicity grades: a Bayesian quasi-likelihood approach. Biometrics **63**(1), 173–179 (2007)

Yuan, Y., Yin, G.: Sequential continual reassessment method for two-dimensional dose finding. Stat. Med. **27**(27), 5664–5678 (2008)

Yuan, Y., Yin, G.: Robust EM continual reassessment method in oncology dose finding. J. Am. Stat. Assoc. **106**(495), 818–831 (2011)

Zhao, L., Lee, J., Mody, R., Braun, T.M.: The superiority of the time-to-event continual reassessment method to the rolling six design in pediatric oncology phase I trials. Clin. Trials **8**(4), 361–369 (2011)

Zhou, Y.: Choosing the number of doses and the cohort size for phase 1 dose-escalation studies. Drug Inf. J. **39**(2), 125–137 (2005)

Zhou, Y., Lucini, M.: Gaining acceptability for the Bayesian decision-theoretic approach in dose-escalation studies. Pharm. Stat. **4**(3), 161–171 (2005)

Zhou, Y., Whitehead, J.: Practical implementation of Bayesian dose-escalation procedures. Drug Inf. J. **37**(1), 45–59 (2003)

Zohar, S., Katsahian, S., O'Quigley, J.: An approach to meta-analysis of dose-finding studies. Stat. Med. **30**(17), 2109–2116 (2011)

Zohar, S., Resche-Rigon, M., Chevret, S.: Using the continual reassessment method to estimate the minimum effective dose in phase II dose-finding studies: a case study. Clin. Trials **10**(3), 414–421 (2013)

Zohar, S., O'Quigley, J.: Sensitivity of dose-finding studies to observation errors. Contemp. Clin. Trials **30**(6), 523–530 (2009)

Chapter 4
Model-Assisted Designs Considering Toxicity Alone

Abstract Phase I trials in oncology are designed to determine the maximum toler-ated doses of agents of interest. The designs can traditionally be classified as rule-/algorithm- or model-based designs. A new design class, known as model-assisted designs, has been developed. In model-assisted designs, the rules of escalation, de-escalation, and maintenance of the current dose are assisted by the model for the toxicity outcome, and are simple and transparent before trial initiation. The model-assisted designs considering toxicity alone include, e.g., the modified toxicity proba-bility interval (mTPI) design and its improved design (the mTPI-2 design), Bayesian optimal interval design, and keyboard design. In this chapter, we overview these designs and discuss related topics.

Keywords Maximum tolerated dose (MTD) · Modified toxicity probability interval (mTPI) design · mTPI-2 design · Bayesian optimal interval (BOIN) design · Keyboard design

4.1 Introduction

Model-assisted designs model the toxicity data at each prespecified dose level, typ-ically using a binomial model. In this regard, this approach is different to that of rule-/algorithm-based designs (see Chap. 2), e.g., the $3 + 3$ design, which only use simple and transparent rules of dose escalation, de-escalation, and maintenance of the current dose. Furthermore, the model-assisted design approach differs from model-based designs (see Chap. 3), e.g., the continual reassessment method (CRM) design, which model a dose–toxicity curve across all doses and continuously update this curve based on data on the administered dose and its corresponding toxicity out-come. Consequently, model-assisted designs have both the simplicity and trans-parency of rule-based designs and the superior performance of model-based designs (Zhou et al. 2018a). Here, "simplicity" means that it is only necessary to count the number of patients experiencing toxicity at the current dose in order to guide the dose escalation, de-escalation, and maintenance. However, the beta-binomial model fitting accompanied by statistical calculation is implicitly required. Further,

T. Daimon et al., *Dose-Finding Designs for Early-Phase Cancer Clinical Trials*, JSS Research Series in Statistics, https://doi.org/10.1007/978-4-431-55585-8_4

81

"transparency" means that the dose escalation, de-escalation, and maintenance rules can be tabulated before trial initiation. Therefore, implementation of model-assisted designs is simpler. In addition, some model-assisted designs exhibit performance comparable to model-based designs. In particular, because model-assisted designs are free from the problem of irrational dose allocation sometimes caused by model mis-specification in model-based designs, they constitute an attractive approach to design of phase I trials (Zhou et al. 2018b). As model-assisted designs considering toxicity alone, there exist, e.g., the modified toxicity probability interval (mTPI) design (Ji et al. 2010), and its improved version (mTPI-2 design) (Guo et al. 2017), the Bayesian optimal interval (BOIN) design (Liu and Yuan 2015), and the keyboard design (Yan et al. 2017). This chapter overviews these designs and discusses related topics.

Unless specifically noted, suppose that the aim of a phase I trial with a prespecified maximum sample size n and target toxicity probability level Γ_T is to identify the MTD of an agent among its increasing ordered doses $d_1 < \ldots < d_K$ corresponding to $1, \ldots, K$ dose levels.

4.2 Modified Toxicity Interval (mTPI) and mTPI-2 Designs

4.2.1 Overview

Ji et al. (2010) presented a modified TPI (mTPI), which is an improved version of "toxicity probability (or posterior) interval (TPI) design", proposed by Ji et al. (2007). One advantage of the mTPI method is that it can be easily understood and implemented by clinical investigators, like the $3+3$ design. This is because the mTPI is algorithmic in that it provides all possible dose assignment actions in advance (Ji and Wang 2013), although it is assisted by a beta-binomial model.

Let π_k be the unknown toxicity probability associated with the kth dose level. Furthermore, π_k is assumed to have a beta prior with hyperparameters α_k and β_k, denoted by $\text{Beta}(\alpha_k, \beta_k)$. For n_k patients treated at dose level k of whom y_k experience toxicity: $\{(n_1, y_1), \ldots, (n_K, y_K)\}$, π_k is assumed to have a beta posterior with hyperparameters $\alpha_k + y_k$ and $\beta_k + n_k - y_k$, denoted by $\text{Beta}(\alpha_k + y_k, \beta_k + n_k - y_k)$ based on the binomial-beta conjugacy. The prior for π_k is usually common and non-informative, because little information is available on the relationship between dose and toxicity in usual phase I trials. Therefore, the prior for π_k is, e.g., $\text{Beta}(0.005, 0.005)$, a U-shaped prior, resulting in a posterior estimate of π_k that is close to the observed toxicity proportion y_k/n_k, or $\text{Beta}(1, 1)$, a flat prior, providing the uniform probability density over $[0, 1]$ (Ji et al. 2007). If a large amount of information is available, one can use a more informative prior.

The mTPI design requires that clinical investigators provide an equivalence interval $[\Gamma_T - \delta_1, \Gamma_T + \delta_2]$ for $\delta_1, \delta_2 (\geq 0)$ close to 0 (say, $\delta_1, \delta_2 = 0.05$), in which the toxicity probability of a given dose level falls if the corresponding dose is close to

Fig. 4.1 An example of the UPMs for three intervals, which are produced by the two vertical lines on the x-axis for the toxicity probability. The UPM for each of the three intervals is given by the dashed horizontal line

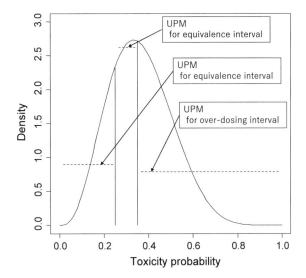

the true MTD. This provides the remaining two intervals: under-donsing interval $(0, \Gamma_T - \delta_1)$, in which the toxicity probability of a given dose level falls if the corresponding dose is below the true MTD, and over-dosing interval $(\Gamma_T + \delta_2, 1)$, in which the toxicity probability falls if the dose level is above the true MTD (see Fig. 4.1). Then, the dose escalation, de-escalation, and maintenance rules of the mTPI design are driven by the unit probability mass (UPM), which is defined as the posterior probability of the toxicity probability falling in each of the aforementioned intervals divided by the length of the corresponding interval. For example, given the data $\{(n_1, y_1), \ldots, (n_K, y_K)\}$ and assuming that π_k has a beta posterior with a cumulative distribution function $\text{Beta}(\pi_k; \alpha', \beta')$, where $\alpha' = \alpha + y_k$ and $\beta' = \beta + n_k - y_k$, the UPM for the equivalence interval $[\Gamma_T - \delta_1, \Gamma_T + \delta_2]$ is given by

$$\text{The UPM for the equivalence interval} = \frac{\text{Beta}(\Gamma_T + \delta_2; \alpha', \beta') - \text{Beta}(\Gamma_T - \delta_1; \alpha', \beta')}{\delta_1 + \delta_2}. \tag{4.1}$$

4.2.2 Dose-Finding Algorithm

The dose-finding algorithm of the mTPI design is given as follows:

Step 1 Treat a patient or cohort of patients at the current dose level $k (\in \{1, \ldots, K\})$, and observe their toxicity outcomes.

Step 2 Calculate the UPMs for the three intervals $(0, \Gamma_T - \delta_1)$, $[\Gamma_T - \delta_1, \Gamma_T + \delta_2]$, and $(\Gamma_T + \delta_2, 1)$ for the current dose level k. Then, escalate to the next highest dose level $k + 1$, retain the current dose level k, or de-escalate to the next lowest dose level $k - 1$, if $(0, \Gamma_T - \delta_1)$, $[\Gamma_T - \delta_1, \Gamma_T + \delta_2]$, or $(\Gamma_T + \delta_2, 1)$ has the largest UPM, respectively.

Step 3 If the maximum sample size is reached, obtain an estimate $\breve{\pi}_k$ of π_k for $k = 1, \ldots, K$, through the isotonic regression procedure of, e.g., Stylianou and Flournoy (2002), while assuming that the toxicity probability increases with the dose level: $0 \leq \pi_1 \leq \ldots \leq \pi_K \leq 1$.

For patient's safety, two additional rules are added to this design. First, suppose that the lowest dose level has been used to treat patients. Given the data $\{(n_1, y_1), \ldots, (n_K, y_K)\}$, calculate the posterior probability of the toxicity probability at the lowest dose level π_1 exceeding Γ_T, $\Pr(\pi_1 > \Gamma_T | n_k, y_k)$. If $\Pr(\pi_1 > \Gamma_T | n_k, y_k) > \xi_1$ for a ξ_1 close to 1 (say, $\xi_1 = 0.95$), terminate the trial due to excessive toxicity. Second, for any dose escalation, if $\Pr(\pi_{k+1} > \Gamma_T) > \xi_2$ for a ξ_2 close to 1 (say, $\xi_2 = 0.95$), retain the dose at level k and exclude dose levels $(k + 1)$ and higher from the trial thereafter.

Risks of underdosing or overdosing are associated with the mTPI design, which are intuitively unacceptable for clinical investigators (see Liu and Yuan (2015), Yang et al. (2015, 2016, 2017), Guo et al. (2017)). For example, as shown by Guo et al. (2017), when the target toxicity probability $\Gamma_T = 0.3$, and three of six patients treated at a certain dose experience toxicity, the mTPI design suggests that the current dose should be retained and more patients should be treated at that dose. Because the empirical toxicity probability is 3/6, or 50%, clinical investigators could argue that the dose should be de-escalated, not retained. Yang et al. (2015) presented an ad hoc remedy that allows the dose escalation, de-escalation, and maintenance rules in the mTPI design to be modified by users. While such an ad hoc remedy provides some flexibility, it becomes difficult to statistically justify the mTPI design.

Guo et al. (2017) indicated that the above suboptimal rules are consequences of the principle of Ockham's razor, which prefers a simple to a complex model if the complex model does not offer a better explanation. To address this issue, they proposed the mTPI-2 design, an extension of the mTPI that blunts the Ockham's razor. Specifically, the mTPI-2 design requires clinical investigators to provide equivalence interval $[\Gamma_T - \delta_1, \Gamma_T + \delta_2]$, like the mTPI design, and then to provide a set of intervals below and above the equivalence interval, dividing the toxicity probability interval $(0, 1)$ into subintervals with equal length of $(\delta_1 + \delta_2)$. This process produces multiple intervals with the same length, which are regarded as multiple equal-sized models. For example, when $\Gamma_T = 0.3$ and $\delta_1 = \delta_2 = 0.05$, the equivalence interval is $[0.25, 0.35]$, and the other intervals are $(0, 0.05)$, $(0.05, 0.15)$, and $(0.15, 0.25)$ below the equivalence interval and $(0.35, 0.45)$, $(0.45, 0.55)$, $(0.55, 0.65)$, $(0.65, 0.75)$, $(0.75, 0.85)$, $(0.85, 0.95)$, and $(0.95, 1)$ above the equivalence interval.

Similar to the mTPI design, if the equivalence interval has the largest UPM, it is selected as the winning model and the mTPI-2 design suggests retention of the dose for treatment of the subsequent patients. If any interval below or above the equivalence dose has the largest UPM, it is selected as the winning model and the mTPI-2 design suggests that the dose should be escalated or de-escalated,

respectively. Therefore, the dose-finding algorithm of the mTPI-2 design is basically the same as that of the mTPI design, except that the three (under-dosing,
proper-dosing, and over-dosing) intervals in the mTPI design are replaced by the
aforementioned set of intervals in the mTPI-2.

4.2.3 Software for Implementation

An Excel macro to implement the mTPI design can be downloaded free of charge at
http://health.bsd.uchicago.edu/yji/software2.htm. Given the maximum sample size
for a trial, the target toxicity probability level, and the equivalence interval, the macro
can tabulate the dose escalation, de-escalation, and maintenance rules in an Excel
spreadsheet. An R program to perform simulations can also be downloaded from the
same site. This program can provide the operating characteristics of the mTPI design
for various scenarios. Another R code for implementing the mTPI design is available
from https://biostatistics.mdanderson.org/softwaredownload/SingleSoftware.aspx?
Software_Id=72. The mTPI-2 design as well as the mTPI design can be implemented through the more user-friendly NextGen-DF, which is a next-generation tool
for design of dose-finding trials in oncology (see Fig. 4.2). This tool allows implementation, comparison, and calibration of several methods via the Web, in real time
and independent of the computer operating system (see Yang et al. (2015)). However,
note that a new Web tool called "U-design", which is an upgrade of NextGen-DF, is
now available at https://udesign.laiyaconsulting.com.

4.3 Keyboard Design

4.3.1 Overview

The keyboard design (Yan et al. 2017) retains the simplicity of the mTPI design,
but avoids its risk of overdosing, achieving higher accuracy identification of the true
MTD. The keyboard design uses a beta-binomial, like the mTPI and mTPI-2 designs.
However, the keyboard design relies on the posterior distribution of the toxicity
probability to guide dose finding, instead of the unit probability mass employed by the
mTPI design. Thus, the former allows for the aforementioned intuitive interpretation,
but the latter does not.

The keyboard design also prespecifies a series of equal-width intervals for the
toxicity probability, called keys, in which the toxicity probability of a given dose
level can fall. Specifically, the keyboard design requires clinical investigators to
provide a proper dosing interval $\mathfrak{I}^* = (\delta_1, \delta_2)$, called the "target key," in which the
true toxicity probability of a given dose level falls if the corresponding dose is close
to the true MTD. Then, investigators must lay a series of keys of equal width on both

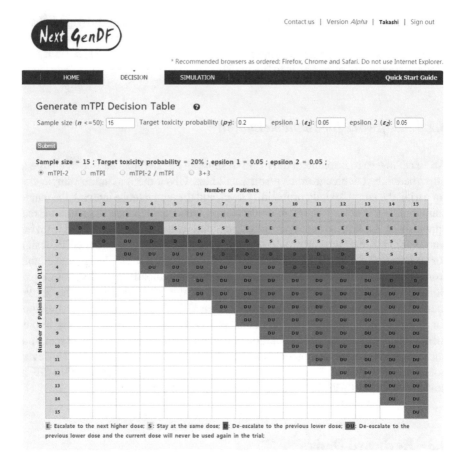

Fig. 4.2 Decision table for dose escalation, de-escalation and maintenance rules for mTPI and mTPI-2 designs

sides of the target key, resulting in a series of I keys of equal width that span the range of 0 to 1, denoted by $\mathfrak{I}_1, \ldots, \mathfrak{I}_I$. For example, for a target key of $(0.15, 0.25)$, nine $(I = 9)$ keys including this target key are laid within the $[0, 1]$ interval with two ends, i.e., <0.05 and >0.95. One key of width 0.1, i.e., $(0.05, 0.15)$ is laid on the left side, whereas 7 keys of width 0.1, i.e., $(0.25, 0.35), \ldots, (0.85, 0.95)$, are laid on the right side. The two ends do not generate problems with regard to dose escalation, de-escalation, and maintenance, although they are not sufficiently wide to form a key.

The keyboard design is equivalent to the mTPI-2 design if the unequally spaced intervals at the lower and upper ends are removed to have equally spaced intervals only in both designs. However, to indicate the most likely location of the true toxicity probability of the current dose level, the former design uses the posterior probability, whereas the latter design uses the unit probability mass on the basis of Ockham's razor. Thus, the keyboard design may be more transparent than the mTPI-2 design.

4.3.2 Dose-Finding Algorithm

The dose-finding algorithm of the keyboard design is given as follows:

Step 1 Treat a patient or cohort of patients at the current dose level $k(\in \{1, \ldots, K\})$ (usually the lowest dose level for the first patient or cohort), and observe their toxicity outcomes.

Step 2 Identify the "strongest key," which has the highest posterior probability, and thus indicates the most likely location of the true toxicity probability of the current dose level. If the strongest key is located on the left side of the target key, meaning that the obtained data on the dose level and toxicity outcome suggest that the current dose level is most likely to be under-dosing, escalate the dose to level $k + 1$. Conversely, if the strongest key is located on the right side of the target, meaning that the data suggests that the current dose level is most likely to be overdosing, de-escalate the dose to level $k - 1$. Finally, if the strongest key is the target key, which means that the data suggest that the current dose level is most likely to be correct dosing, maintain the current dose.

Step 3 If the maximum sample size is reached, obtain an estimate of the toxicity probability through an isotonic regression procedure and then identify this dose as the MTD.

For patient's safety, a rule of dose elimination is added to this design. If the obtained data on the dose level and toxicity outcome indicate that there is a greater than 95% chance that the current dose is above the MTD, that is, $\Pr(\pi_k \geq \Gamma_T | n_k, y_k) > 0.95$, the current dose and higher dose levels are eliminated from the trial. However, before the dose elimination rule is applied, a minimum of three patients have to be evaluated.

4.3.3 Software for Implementation

To implement the Keyboard design, a Shiny application with detailed instructions and templates for protocol preparation is available at http://www.trialdesign.org/. If the number of doses, the starting dose level, the target toxicity probability level, the toxicity probability interval, the cohort size, the cohort number, and the cutoff for overdose control are supplied, we can obtain a decision table for dose escalation and de-escalation for the keyboard design (see Fig. 4.3).

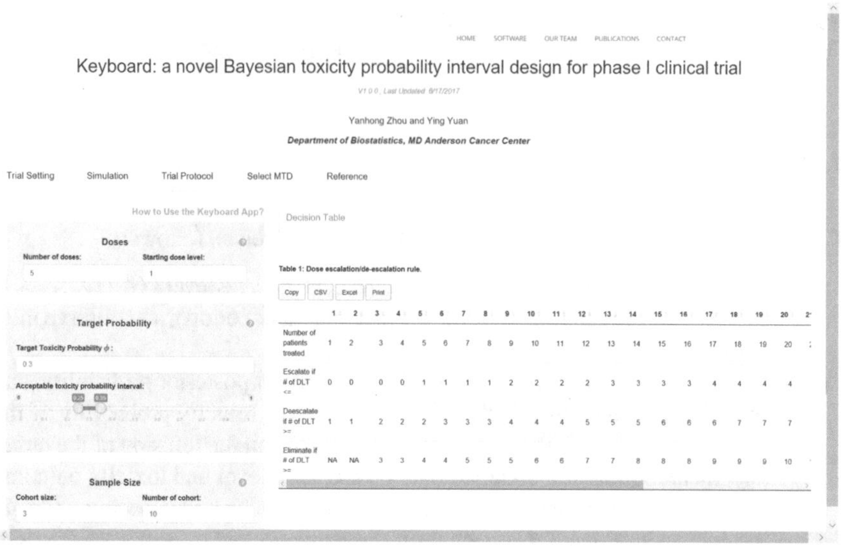

Fig. 4.3 Decision table for dose escalation and de-escalation for keyboard design

4.4 Bayesian Optimal Interval Designs

4.4.1 Overview

Liu and Yuan (2015) proposed the local and general Bayesian optimal interval (BOIN) designs for MTD identification, which are intended to minimize the chance of exposing patients to subtherapeutic or overly toxic doses. Liu and Yuan (2015) recommend use of the local BOIN design, because finite-sample simulations suggest that the local BOIN design has better performance than the general BOIN design. Thus, in the following, we focus on the local BOIN design, and hereafter simply call the local BOIN design as "the BOIN design". The BOIN design is more straightforward and transparent than the aforementioned model-assisted designs. In fact, the BOIN design provides dose escalation, de-escalation, and maintenance suggestions in a easy-to-understand manner, by comparing the estimated toxicity probability at the current dose level with a pair of fixed dose escalation and de-escalation boundaries.

4.4.2 Dose-Finding Algorithm

Let π_k denote the true toxicity probability of dose level k for $k = 1, \ldots, K$. Based on data that n_k patients were treated at dose level k and y_k of them experienced toxicity, the toxicity probability at the current dose is estimated by $\hat{\pi}_k = y_k/n_k$. Further, let $\lambda_{1k}(n_k, \Gamma_T)$ and $\lambda_{2k}(n_k, \Gamma_T)$ denote the precalculated dose escalation and de-escalation boundaries, respectively.

The dose-finding algorithm of the BOIN design is given as follows:

Step 1 Treat a patient or cohort of patients at the current dose level $k(\in \{1, \ldots, K\})$ (usually the lowest dose level for the first patient or cohort), and observe their toxicity outcomes.

Step 2 Estimate the toxicity probability at the current dose level. If $\hat{\pi}_k \leq \lambda_{T,1}(n_k, \Gamma_T)$, escalate the dose to level $k + 1$; if $\hat{\pi}_k \geq \lambda_{T,2}(n_k, \Gamma_T)$, de-escalate the dose to level $k - 1$; otherwise, maintain the dose at the current dose level.

Step 3 If the maximum sample size is reached, obtain an estimate of the toxicity probability through an isotonic regression procedure and then identify the MTD.

Similar to the keyboard design, for patient's safety, a dose elimination rule is added to the BOIN design.

The BOIN design is based on three-point hypotheses: H_0 indicates that the current dose is therapeutic and, thus, dose retention should be performed to treat the next cohort of patients; H_1 indicates that the current dose is subtherapeutic and, thus, dose escalation should be performed; and H_2 indicates that the current dose is toxic and, thus, dose escalation should be performed. Note that these three hypotheses are not specified with the aim of representing the truth and testing the hypotheses, but rather to optimize the performance of this design.

The three-point hypotheses are formulated for π_k as follows:

$$H_{0k} : \pi_k = \Gamma_T, \quad H_{1k} : \pi_k = \Gamma_{T,1}, \text{ and } H_{2k} : \pi_k = \Gamma_{T,2}, \tag{4.2}$$

where $\Gamma_{T,1}$ denotes the highest toxicity probability level considered to be below the MTD and $\Gamma_{T,2}$ denotes the lowest toxicity probability level considered to be above the MTD. To minimize the probability of incorrectly deciding the dose assignment, $\lambda_{1k}(n_k, \Gamma_T)$ and $\lambda_{2k}(n_k, \Gamma_T)$ are determined as follows:

$$\lambda_{1k}(n_k, \Gamma_T) = \frac{\log\left(\frac{1 - \Gamma_{T,1}}{1 - \Gamma_T}\right) + n_j^{-1} \log\left(\frac{\Pr(H_{1k})}{\Pr(H_{0k})}\right)}{\log\left(\frac{\Gamma_T(1 - \Gamma_{T,1})}{\Gamma_{T,1}(1 - \Gamma_T)}\right)},$$

$$\lambda_{2k}(n_k, \Gamma_T) = \frac{\log\left(\frac{1 - \Gamma_T}{1 - \Gamma_{T,2}}\right) + n_j^{-1} \log\left(\frac{\Pr(H_{0k})}{\Pr(H_{2k})}\right)}{\log\left(\frac{\Gamma_{T,2}(1 - \Gamma_T)}{\Gamma(1 - \Gamma_{T,2})}\right)}.$$

When $\Pr(H_{0k}) = \Pr(H_{1k}) = \Pr(H_{3k})$, $\lambda_{1k}(n_k, \Gamma_T)$ and $\lambda_{2k}(n_k, \Gamma_T)$ are invariant to both dose level k and the corresponding sample size n_k. The invariance property simplifies the trial conduct because the same pair of interval boundaries can be used during the trial regardless of k and n_k.

4.4.3 Software for Implementation

Software to implement the BOIN designs are available as the "BOIN" R package from https://cran.r-project.org/web/packages/BOIN/index.html, as a standalone graphical user interface-based Windows desktop program from https://biostatistics.mdanderson.org/softwaredownload/SingleSoftware.aspx?Software_Id=99, and as Shiny online applications from http://www.trialdesign.org/. For example, given the target toxicity probability level, the cohort size, and the number of cohorts, as necessary, the early stopping parameter, the highest toxicity probability considered to be subtherapeutic (i.e., below the MTD) such that dose escalation should be performed, the lowest toxicity probability considered overly toxic such that de-escalation is required, and the cutoff to eliminate an overly toxic dose for safety, we can obtain the dose escalation and de-escalation boundaries using the function get.boundary in the BOIN R package:

```
get.boundary(target=0.3, ncohort=8, cohortsize=3)

$`lambda_e`
[1] 0.2364907

$lambda_d
[1] 0.3585195

$boundary_tab

Number of patients treated 3  6  9 12 15 18 21 24
Escalate if # of DLT <=     0  1  2  2  3  4  4  5
Deescalate if # of DLT >=   2  3  4  5  6  7  8  9
Eliminate if # of DLT >=    3  4  5  7  8  9 10 11

$full_boundary_tab

Number of patients treated  1  2  3  4  5  6  7  8  9 10 11 12 13
Escalate if # of DLT <=      0  0  0  0  1  1  1  1  2  2  2  2  3
Deescalate if # of DLT >=    1  1  2  2  2  3  3  3  4  4  4  5  5
Eliminate if # of DLT >=    NA NA  3  3  4  4  5  5  5  6  6  7  7

Number of patients treated 14 15 16 17 18 19 20 21 22 23 24
Escalate if # of DLT <=      3  3  3  4  4  4  4  4  5  5  5
Deescalate if # of DLT >=    6  6  6  7  7  7  8  8  8  9  9
Eliminate if # of DLT >=     8  8  8  9  9  9 10 10 11 11 11
```

4.5 A New Class of Dose-Finding Designs

Clertant and O'Quigley (2017) described a new class of dose-finding design, i.e., semiparametric dose-finding designs, for phase I trials. Under some parametric conditions, this class reduces to the family of CRM designs. However, if the underlying structure is relaxed, this class encompasses the cumulative cohort, mTPI, and BOIN designs, which do not explicitly model a dose–toxicity curve under a single umbrella. For details, see Clertant and O'Quigley (2017) and for further discussions, the readers are referred to Clertant and O'Quigley (2019). The R code is available from https://github.com/MatthieuMC/SPM_project_01.

4.6 The Best Design?

Horton et al. (2017) compared the mTPI, BOIN, and CRM designs in a simulation study with 16 dose–toxicity relationship scenarios. They showed that, when the correct selection rate for the true MTD and the dose allocation accuracy are considered, the CRM design outperforms the other two designs in most scenarios, followed by BOIN and then mTPI. Furthermore, these trends are more notable as the number of dose levels is increased.

Ananthakrishnan et al. (2017) investigated rule-based designs, including $3 + 3$, $A + B$, $3 + 3 + 3$, and accelerated titration designs; model-based designs, including the CRM and escalation with overdose control (EWOC) designs; and model-assisted designs, including mTPI, BOIN, and frequentist versions of mTPI called toxicity equivalence range (TEQR) designs, using three dose–toxicity relationship scenarios. They showed that the $5 + 5a$ design selects the MTD with equivalent accuracy to the model-based and model-assisted designs for the linear and log-logistic dose–toxicity relationship scenarios, but requires enrollment of a higher number of patients. In addition, the model-based and model-assisted designs perform well and give the highest accuracy for dose allocation, and also have a reasonably high proportion of true MTD selection.

Zhou et al. (2018a) reviewed model-assisted designs such as the mTPI, keyboard, and BOIN designs, and compared their performance with the CRM design, based on 10,000 dose–toxicity relationship scenarios randomly generated by the pseudo-uniform algorithm proposed by Clertant and O'Quigley (2017). Their results show that the BOIN, keyboard, and CRM designs provide comparable superior operating characteristics, and that each outperforms the mTPI design. Zhou et al. (2018b) reviewed three model-assisted designs, including the mTPI, BOIN, and keyboard designs, and three model-based designs, including the CRM, EWOC, and Bayesian logistic regression model (BLRM), and investigated their accuracy, safety, and reliability. They also considered the empirical rules used in some designs, such as dose skipping and imposition of overdose control. The results show that the CRM design outperforms the EWOC and BLRM designs in terms of MTD identification accuracy, and that the BOIN and keyboard designs have similar performance, outperforming the mTPI. Furthermore, the CRM and BOIN designs have competitive performance.

Clertant and O'Quigley (2019) provided semiparametric extensions for each of the cumulative cohort design (see Sect. 2.9), and the aforementioned model-assisted designs, called "SP-CCD", "SP-MTPI", "SP-BOIN", and "SP-Keyboard", and through extensive simulations, showed that each of these designs improves the performance of the corresponding original design.

4.7 Overview of Other Designs with Related Topics

4.7.1 Designs for Time-to-Toxicity Outcome

Lin and Yin (2017a, b) developed a nonparametric overdose control (NOC) phase I trial design, based on the Bayesian model selection paradigm. In addition, to address the late-onset toxicity issue, they proposed a fractional NOC design that combines the NOC design with the so-called fractional imputation method. These NOC designs can control the posterior probability that each successive dose allocation exceeds the MTD with no assumption of a dose–toxicity curve. R codes to implement the NOC designs are available from Github, at https://github.com/ruitaolin/NOC.

Yuan et al. (2018) proposed the time-to-event BOIN (TITE-BOIN) design for phase I trials with a time-to-toxicity outcome. This design allows real-time dose assignment decisions for new patients while toxicity data for some enrolled patients remain unavailable. Like the BOIN design, the TITE-BOIN dose escalation, de-escalation, and maintenance rules can also be tabulated before trial initiation. Thus, this design is transparent and simple to implement. Compared with the time-to-event continuous reassessment method (TITE-CRM), the TITE-BOIN has comparable MTD identification accuracy, but simpler implementation and substantially better overdose control. The TITE-BOIN design is available as a stand-alone graphical user interface-based Windows desktop program from https://biostatistics.mdanderson. org/softwaredownload/SingleSoftware.aspx?Software_Id=99, or at http://www.trial design.org/.

4.7.2 Designs for Ordinal or Continuous Toxicity Outcomes

Mu et al. (2019) developed a generalized BOIN (gBOIN) design that accommodates toxicity grades or binary or continuous toxicity outcomes under a unified paradigm. The gBOIN design provides the dose escalation, de-escalation, and maintenance rules, based on the exponential family of distributions. The gBOIN design is available at http://www.trialdesign.org/.

4.7.3 Designs for Drug Combinations

Lin and Yin (2017a, b) developed a BOIN design for drug combination trials, for which the dose allocation rule is based on maximization of the posterior probability that the toxicity probability of the next dose falls within a prespecified probability interval. They showed that the proposed design has comparable performance with model-based designs. This is available as a stand-alone graphical user interface-based Windows desktop program at https://biostatistics.mdanderson.org/softwaredownload/SingleSoftware.aspx?Software_Id=99, or at http://www.trialdesign.org/.

Pan et al. (2017) extended the keyboard design for drug combination dose-finding trials. They evaluated the performance of the proposed keyboard design using a generating algorithm for a random two-dimensional dose–toxicity relationship scenario. Their results show that the keyboard design for drug combination generally outperforms the partial order CRM (Wages et al. 2011) in terms of MTD identification accuracy and treatment efficiency. This design is available at http://www.trialdesign.org/.

Mander and Sweeting (2015) proposed a product of independent beta probabilities escalation (PIPE) design to determine the MTD contour based on Bayesian model averaging for drug combination trials, in which no dose–toxicity model is assumed. Zhang and Yuan (2016) also developed the "waterfall" design to determine the MTD contour for drug combination trials. The term "waterfall" represents the process of sequential the MTD contour finding, through moving from the top of the dose matrix to the bottom. As a consequence, this design partitions the dose matrix into subtrials, and the subtrials are conducted using the BOIN design. The waterfall design can be implemented using the "BOIN" R package, which is available from https://cran.r-project.org/web/packages/BOIN/index.html. For further discussion of drug combination trial design, readers are referred to Yuan and Zhang (2017).

References

Ananthakrishnan, R., Green, S., Chang, M., Doros, G., Massaro, J., LaValley, M.: Systematic comparison of the statistical operating characteristics of various phase I oncology designs. Contemp. Clin. Trials Commun. **5**, 34–48 (2017)

Clertant, M., O'Quigley, J.: Semiparametric dose finding methods. J. Roy. Stat. Soc. Ser. B Stat. Methodol. **79**(5), 1487–1508 (2017)

Clertant, M., O'Quigley, J.: Semiparametric dose finding methods: special cases. J. R. Stat. Soc. Ser. C Appl. Stat. **68**(2), 271–288 (2019)

Guo, W., Wang, S.-J., Yang, S., Lin, S., Ji, Y.: A Bayesian interval dose-finding design addressing Ockham's razor: mTPI-2. Comtemp. Clin. Trials **58**, 23–33 (2017)

Horton, B.J., Wages, N.A., Conaway, M.R.: Performance of toxicity probability interval based designs in contrast to the continual reassessment method. Stat. Med. **36**(2), 291–300 (2017)

Ji, Y., Li, Y., Bekele, B.N.: Dose-finding in phase I clinical trials based on toxicity probability interval. Clin. Trials **4**(3), 235–244 (2007)

Ji, Y., Liu, P., Li, Y., Bekele, B.N.: A modified toxicity probability interval method for dose-finding trials. Clin. Trials **7**(6), 653–663 (2010)

Ji, Y., Wang, S.: Modified toxicity probability interval design: a safer and more reliable method than the 3 + 3 design for practical phase I trials. J. Clin. Oncol. **31**(14), 1785–1791 (2013)

Lin, R., Yin, G.: Nonparametric overdose control with late-onset toxicity in phase I clinical trials. Biostatistics **18**(1), 180–194 (2017b)

Lin, R., Yin, G.: Bayesian optimal interval designs for dose finding in drug-combination trials. Stat. Methods Med. Res. **26**(5), 2155–2167 (2017a)

Liu, S., Yuan, Y.: Bayesian optimal interval designs for phase I clinical trials. J. Roy. Stat. Soc. Ser. C Appl. Stat. **64**(3), 507–523 (2015)

Mander, A.P., Sweeting, M.J.: A product of independent beta probabilities dose escalation design for dual-agent phase I trials. Stat. Med. **34**(8), 1261–1276 (2015)

Mu, R., Yuan, Y., Xu, J., Mandrekar, S.J., Yin, J.: gBOIN: a unified model-assisted phase I trial design accounting for toxicity grades, binary or continuous end points. J. R. Stat. Soc. Ser. C Appl. Stat. **68**(2), 289–308 (2019)

Pan, H., Lin, R., Yuan, Y.: Statistical properties of the keyboard design with extension to drug-combination trials (2017). http://arxiv.org/abs/1712.06718

Stylianou, M., Flournoy, N.: Dose finding using the biased coin up-and-down design and isotonic regression. Biometrics **58**(1), 171–177 (2002)

Wages, N.A., Conaway, M.R., O'Quigley, J.: Continual reassessment method for partial ordering. Biometrics **67**(4), 1555–1563 (2011)

Yan, F., Mandrekar, S.J., Yuan, Y.: Keyboard: a novel Bayesian toxicity probability interval design for phase I clinical trials. Clin. Cancer Res. **23**(15), 3994–4003 (2017)

Yang, S., Wang, S.-J., Ji, Y.: An integrated dose-finding tool for phase I trials in oncology. Contemp. Clin. Trials **45**(Part B), 426–434 (2015)

Yuan, Y., Hess, K.R., Hilsenbeck, S.G., Gilbert, M.R.: Bayesian optimal interval design: a simple and well-performing design for phase I oncology trials. Clin. Cancer Res. **22**(17), 4291–4301 (2016)

Yuan, Y., Lin, R., Li, D., Nie, L., Warren, K.E.: Time-to-event Bayesian optimal interval design to accelerate phase I trials. Clin. Cancer Res. **24**(20), 4921–4930 (2018)

Yuan, Y., Zhang, L.: Chapter 6. Designing early-phase drug combination trials. In: O'Quigley J., Iasonos, A., Bornkamp, B. (eds.) Handbook of Methods for Designing, Monitoring, and Analyzing Dose Finding Trials, 1st edn., pp. 109–126 (2017)

Zhang, L., Yuan, Y.: A practical Bayesian design to identify the maximum tolerated dose contour for drug combination trials. Stat. Med. **35**(27), 4924–4936 (2016)

Zhou, H., Murray, T.A., Pan, H., Yuan, Y.: Comparative review of novel model-assisted designs for phase I clinical trials. Stat. Med. (2018a). https://doi.org/10.1002/sim.7674

Zhou, H., Yuan, Y., Nie, L.: Accuracy, safety, and reliability of novel phase I trial designs. Clin. Cancer Res. **24**(18), 4357–4364 (2018b)

Chapter 5
Designs Considering Toxicity and Efficacy

Abstract The primary objective of a phase I trial is conventionally to determine the maximum tolerated dose (MTD) of a new agent, on the premise that its toxicity and efficacy monotonically increase with increasing dose. This is because the MTD is expected to produce maximal efficacy under admissible toxicity; thus, this dose is basically adopted as the optimal dose in the subsequent phase II and III trials. However, this paradigm is not necessarily suitable for a cytostatic, molecularly targeted, or biological agent. In addition, for any agents, the true relationship among dose, toxicity, and efficacy cannot be known. Therefore, to address these issues, the so-called "phase I/II," which combines a phase I trial and a phase II trial into one trial, may be helpful in considering both efficacy and toxicity. This chapter overviews several rule-based, model-based, and model-assisted designs for such trials, and discusses related topics.

Keywords Phase I/II trial · Rule-based designs · Model-based designs · Model-assisted designs

5.1 Introduction

For chemotherapeutic agents (CAs) or cytotoxic agents, there is a presupposition that toxicity and efficacy monotonically increase with dose. This is because the mechanisms of action of such agents with regard to both toxicity and efficacy are basically the same. As a consequence, the dose–efficacy relationship is parallel with the dose–toxicity relationship, with each behaving as a monotonically increasing function of the dose. Thus, the therapeutic effect is predictable on the basis of the dose intensity for the toxic effect. Anticipating such a presupposition or consequence, various phase I trial designs focused on evaluation of toxicity alone have been applied in practice, as discussed in Chaps. 2–4.

However, for patients participating in an agent trial or future patients who will receive this agent as a drug in practice, if a certain dose is admissible with regard to toxicity but yields low or no efficacy, the dose or agent itself is essentially useless. In addition, unlike most CAs or cytotoxic agents, cytostatic agents, MTAs, or IAs, for example, do not always present a parallel relationship between dose–toxicity and dose–efficacy with monotonic increases in dose, because of their specific mechanisms of action. In fact, some of these agents can have weaker or slight toxicity. In such cases, emphasis should be placed on efficacy evaluation rather than toxicity evaluation, although unfortunately, the phase I trial designs considering toxicity alone (see Chaps. 2–4) have often been used in practice, sometimes including dose expansion cohorts (see Sect. 6.5). As a consequence, the trial may take the form of a simultaneous or seamless combination of a phase I trial with a phase II trial. Such a trial is conducted as a so-called "phase I/II or I–II trial." Because the terms "phase I/II trial" and "phase I–II trial" are used interchangeably, we simply call them as "phase I/II trial." In this chapter, we overview some phase I/II trial designs.

5.2   What Is the Optimal Dose?

Suppose that, in a phase I/II trial with a prespecified maximum sample size n_{max}, clinical investigators attempt to identify the optimal dose (OD) for an agent among the ordered doses $d_1 < \cdots < d_K$, where the toxicity and efficacy outcomes are both observed as a binary outcome. Let X denote the random variable for a dose administered to a patient enrolled in the trial, and x an observed value as $x \in \{d_1, \ldots, d_K\}$. Let Y_T denote the random variable for the binary toxicity outcome and y_T denote an observed value of Y_T, where $Y_T = 1$ indicates toxicity and $Y_T = 0$ otherwise. Similarly, let Y_E denote the random variable for the binary efficacy outcome and y_E denote an observed value of Y_T, where $Y_E = 1$ indicates efficacy and $Y_E = 0$ otherwise. We denote the probability of Y_T, probability of Y_E, and bivariate probability of Y_T and Y_E given dose x as follows:

$$\Pr(Y_T = y_T | X = x), \ y_T \in \{0, 1\}, \tag{5.1}$$

$$\Pr(Y_E = y_E | X = x), \ y_E \in \{0, 1\}, \tag{5.2}$$

and

$$\Pr(Y_T = y_T, Y_E = y_E | X = x), \ y_T, y_E \in \{0, 1\}, \tag{5.3}$$

where if Y_T and Y_E are assumed to be independent, $\Pr(Y_T = y_T, Y_E = y_E | X = x) = \Pr(Y_T = y_T | X = x)\Pr(Y_E = y_E | X = x)$.

Let Γ_T denote the prespecified target toxicity probability level or maximum admissible toxicity probability level for $\Pr(Y_T = 1 | X = x)$. From the perspective of toxicity, an admissible dose is defined as a dose that satisfies the relation.

$$\Pr(Y_T = 1 | X = x) \leq \Gamma_T. \tag{5.4}$$

As shown in Chaps. 2–4, the primary objective of phase I trials, especially for cytotoxic agents, is to determine the maximum tolerated dose (MTD), where the maximum dose is selected as the MTD among the admissible doses that satisfy Eq. (5.4). The MTD is regarded as the OD if the toxicity and efficacy increase monotonically and in parallel with the increasing dose.

Let Γ_E denote the prespecified minimum efficacy probability level for $\Pr(Y_E = 1|X = x)$. From the perspective of efficacy, an admissible dose is defined as the dose that satisfies the relation.

$$\Pr(Y_E = 1|X = x) \geq \Gamma_E. \tag{5.5}$$

In some trials, the goal may be to determine the minimum effective dose (MED) that produces a therapeutic response or desired effect in some fraction of the patients receiving the agent. In such trials, the minimum dose is selected as the MED from among the admissible doses that satisfy Eq. (5.5).

In some phase I/II trials for patients with serious diseases and life-threatening illnesses, because toxicity is fatal, the efficacy outcome is censored. In such cases, because the marginal distribution of the efficacy outcome cannot be obtained, the toxicity and efficacy outcomes can be reduced to the trinomial outcome (Thall and Russell 1998): $(Y_T, Y_E) = (0, 0)$, $(Y_T, Y_E) = (0, 1)$, and $Y_T = 1$. Of the trinomial outcomes, $(Y_T, Y_E) = (0, 1)$ can be the most desirable. The occurrence of such an outcome is often referred to as "success." Then, for the probability of success $\Pr(Y_T = 0, Y_E = 1|X = x)$, the MED in Eq. (5.5) may be instead defined as the minimum dose that satisfies the relation.

$$\Pr(Y_T = 0, Y_E = 1|X = x) \geq \Gamma_E. \tag{5.6}$$

For these probabilities, let us define the following functions of dose x, i.e., the dose–toxicity, dose–efficacy, and dose–success curves, $R(x)$, $Q(x)$, and $P(x)$, respectively:

$$R(x) = \Pr(Y_T = 1|X = x), \tag{5.7}$$

$$Q(x) = \Pr(Y_E = 1|X = x), \tag{5.8}$$

and

$$P(x) = \Pr(Y_T = 0, Y_E = 1|X = x). \tag{5.9}$$

Again, if Y_T and Y_E are assumed to be independent, $P(x)$ can be given by $P(x) = Q(x)\{1 - R(x)\}$.

The primary objective of phase I/II trials is to determine the dose with the highest admissible efficacy together with admissible toxicity. Then, a dose that maximizes $\Pr(Y_T = 0, Y_E = 1|X = x)$ while meeting threshold Γ_E in Eq. (5.6) can be considered. This dose is sometimes called the "OD," the "most successful dose (MSD)," etc. (see Ivanova 2003, Zohar and O'Quigley 2006a, and Zohar and O'Quigley 2006b). This dose is also sometimes required to satisfy Eqs. (5.4) and (5.5) or (5.6). This dose is sometimes called the "optimal safe dose (OSD)," "the safe MSD," etc. (see Ivanova 2003, Zohar and O'Quigley 2006a, and Zohar and O'Quigley 2006b).

5.3   Rule-Based Designs

Gooley et al. (1994) investigated rule-based designs for a bone marrow transplantation trial incorporating two competing outcomes; that is, graft-versus-host-disease
and no rejection. These two competing outcomes can be considered as toxicity and
efficacy outcomes in our context, that is, Y_T and Y_E, respectively, which are assumed
to be independent. Those researchers showed the importance and benefits of simulation for evaluation of the operating characteristics of a proposed design. Note that
there were no explicit models for dose–outcome relationships, although it is assumed
that they were monotonic in dose x. The goal of the trial was to determine admissible doses satisfying both Eqs. (5.4) and (5.5). Through simulations, several different
designs were investigated. With this research as a starting point, many rule-based,
model-based, or model-assisted designs have been developed. In the following, we
describe some of them for phase I/II trials.

5.3.1   Optimizing Up-and-Down Design

Kpamegan and Flournoy (2001) proposed a phase I/II optimizing up-and-down
design (see Sect. 2.3) to treat more subjects at the OD. Here, the OD can be considered
as the dose that aims to maximize $\Pr(Y_T = 0, Y_E = 1|X = x)$ in Eq. (5.6).

The dose-finding algorithm requires that patients are treated in pairs with adjacent
doses. The first pair of patients is treated at doses (d_1, d_2). Suppose that the most
recent pair of patients is treated at doses (d_k, d_{k+1}), $k \in \{k = 1, \ldots, K - 1\}$. The
next pair of patients is treated at

1. doses (d_{k-1}, d_k), if the patient treated at dose d_k has experienced success, the
   patient treated at dose d_{k+1} has experienced no success, and $k > 1$;
2. doses (d_{k+1}, d_{k+2}), if the patient treated at dose d_{k+1} has experienced success, the
   patient treated at dose d_k has experienced no success, and $k + 1 < K$; and
3. doses (d_k, d_{k+1}) otherwise.

For the lowest and highest doses, this design makes appropriate adjustments, such that
it treats the pair at (d_1, d_2) instead of (d_0, d_1), and (d_{K-1}, d_K) instead of (d_K, d_{K+1}).

5.3.2   Play-the-Winner-Like Design

Ivanova (2003) proposed a phase I/II design to find the OSD that maximizes the
success probability subject to the toxicity restriction, where success is defined as the
joint event of the presence of efficacy and the lack of toxicity. Because of the toxicity
restriction, focus is placed on the doses for which the toxicity probability does not
exceed the maximum admissible toxicity level (see Sect. 5.2). This design is based

on the play-the-winner rule (Zelen 1969) in that it continues to treat patients at the dose that yields success.

The first patient is treated at dose d_1. Suppose that the most recent patient is treated at dose d_k, $k \in \{1, \ldots, K\}$. For the next patient,

1. de-escalate the dose to d_{k-1}, if the most recent patient has experienced toxicity;
2. remain at d_k, if the most recent patient has experienced success; and
3. escalate the dose to d_{k+1}, if the most recent patient has experienced no toxicity and no efficacy.

For the lowest and highest doses, this design makes appropriate adjustments, such that the patient is treated at d_1 instead of d_0, and d_K instead of d_{K+1}.

Ivanova (2003) demonstrated that the mode of stationary treatment distribution is close to or coincides with the OSD. In addition, that author presented some practical considerations, such as modifications of the cohort size, stopping rules, and OSD estimation.

5.3.3 Directed-Walk Designs

Hardwick et al. (2003) proposed designs that combine directed walks with smoothed shape-constrained fitting to dose–outcome curves, for the problem of OD identification. These directed walks are related to random walks, but are not constrained by the Markov assumption. As a consequence, all available information can be used to determine each dose allocation, as discussed below.

For dose x, $R(x)$ (see Eq. 5.7), $Q(x)$ (see Eq. 5.8), and $P(x)$ (see Eq. 5.9) are considered, where $R(x)$ and $Q(x)$ are assumed to be independent of each other and nondecreasing in dose x. Further, $P(x)$ is given by $P(x) = Q(x) \{1 - R(x)\}$. However, $Q(x)$ cannot always be defined, because the efficacy is censored when the toxicity is severe, as discussed by, e.g., Thall and Russell (1998), Kpamegan and Flournoy (2001), and O'Quigley et al. (2001). To address this issue, Hardwick et al. (2003) also replaced Q with the following dose–efficacy curve, given the absence of a toxic response:

$$Q'(x) = \Pr(Y_E = 1 | Y_X = 0, X = x), \tag{5.10}$$

and redefine the probability of success as

$$P'(x) = Q'(x) \{1 - R(x)\}. \tag{5.11}$$

In these cases, it is assumed that $Q'(x)$ is nondecreasing and that $P'(x)$ is unimodal. This assumption of unimodality of the dose–success curve helps ensure estimator consistency. In cases in which $P'(x)$ is unimodal but $P(x)$ is insteadly utilized, because the dependency structure between efficacy and toxicity is unknown, the designs can target the mode location, provided $P'(x)$ is a monotonic function of $P(x)$. Then, the dose with the mode is taken as the OD. The $R(x)$ and $Q(x)$ curves are estimated independently using the data on previous dose assignments and outcomes, and the dose allocated to the next patient is based on the estimated OD location. To guide the dose-finding algorithm in these designs, Hardwick et al. (2003) explored the parametric or nonparametric methods for estimation of the curves, as well as the maximum likelihood, smoothed maximum likelihood estimation, or Bayesian estimators.

In the following, we mainly outline the start-up procedure and some nonparametric methods for the curve fitting and estimation. The start-up procedure of these designs is used to allow for the curve fitting and estimation. This is true for maximum likelihood estimators, but not for Bayesian estimators (see Sect. 3.2.2.2). Specifically, depending on the curve-fitting method, the dose-finding algorithm may adhere to the following up-and-down design (see Sect. 2.3): If $(Y_T, Y_E) = (0, 0)$, escalate the dose; if $(Y_T, Y_E) = (0, 1)$, remain at the current dose; if $(Y_T, Y_E) = (1, 1)$, de-escalate the dose; and if $(Y_T, Y_E) = (1, 0)$, apply an exploration procedure (for details, Hardwick et al. 2003). The dose-finding algorithm can be initiated at any dose, terminates the trial after n_{max} patients have been treated, and estimates the OD according to either of the following curve-estimation methods or other techniques. If the data are not sufficient for the curve estimation, the dose that provides the highest observed success rate is chosen.

Seven methods to model the dose–toxicity and dose–efficacy relationships and to obtain estimators for the dose–success relationship on some fixed set of dose levels $\{d_1, \ldots, d_K\}$ have been examined by Hardwick et al. (2003). Here, we focus on four nonparametric shape-constrained methods. Suppose that $x \in \{d_1, \ldots, d_K\}$ and that the data for the first j included patients $\mathfrak{D}_j = \{(x_l, y_{T,l}, y_{E,l}); l = 1, \ldots, j\}$ $(j = 1, \ldots, n_{max})$ are obtained. Focusing on the toxicity data in $\mathfrak{D}_j$, j_k observations at dose level d_k have been performed, which are classified as $j_{k,0}$ toxic and $(j_k - j_{k,0})$ nontoxic responses. Then, the binomial likelihood function for the toxicity outcome is given by

$$\prod_{k=1}^{K} \binom{j_k}{j_{k,0}} \{R(d_k)\}^{j_{k,0}} \{1 - R(d_k)\}^{j_k - j_{k,0}} . \tag{5.12}$$

For the efficacy outcome, Q can be substituted for R.

The nonparametric approaches are described as follows:

Convex–concave.   A shape-constrained maximum likelihood estimator maximizes the likelihood under shape assumptions of Q.

Smoothed convex–concave.   A term is added to the likelihood (5.12) to penalize smoothness:

$$\prod_{k=1}^{K} \binom{j_k}{j_{k,0}} \{R(d_k)\}^{j_{k,0}} \{1 - R(d_k)\}^{j_k - j_{k,0}} \prod_{k=2}^{K} \left(\frac{R(d_k) - R(d_{k-1})}{d_k - d_{k-1}} \right)^{\lambda} , \tag{5.13}$$

where λ is the smoothing parameter.

Monotone.   For each dose k such that $j_k > 0$, let $\hat{R}(d_k) = j_{k,0}/j_k$ denote the observed toxicity rate. The monotone shape-constrained maximum likelihood estimator is obtained from the weighted least-squares monotone regression of $\hat{R}(d_k)$, where $\hat{R}(d_k)$ is weighted by j_k.

Smoothed monotone.   The probability toxicity at each dose is assumed to have a beta prior. For every enrolled patient, a weighted least-squares monotone regression is applied.

Hardwick et al. (2003) explored designs that perform well along two performance measures: a sampling efficiency to assess experimental losses and a decision efficiency to predict future losses on the basis of the final decision.

5.3.4 Odds-Ratio Trade-off Design

Yin et al. (2006) proposed a Bayesian phase I/II trial design to consider the bivariate toxicity and efficacy outcomes of an agent, where the bivariate binary toxicity and efficacy data are jointly modeled to account for the association between them, without specification of any parametric function for the dose–outcome curves. In addition, the toxicity–efficacy odds-ratio trade-off is considered for dose allocation.

For dose $x \in \{d_1, \ldots, d_K\}$, it is assumed that $R(x)$ monotonically increases, but $Q(x)$ has no monotonic constraint. This assumption may be reasonable for some cytostatic agents, MTAs, or IAs, because the efficacy may not always increase as the dose increases. Note that, because no parametric models to account for the inter-dose dependency are specified, this design can be regarded as rule based in our context. Yin et al. (2006) used a global cross-ratio (Dale 1986) as an association measure suitable for bivariate, discrete, or ordered outcomes. This global cross-ratio model can be considered for the bivariate outcomes at dose level k as follows:

$$\beta_k = \frac{\Pr(Y_T = 0, Y_E = 0|X = d_k)\Pr(Y_T = 1, Y_E = 1|X = d_k)}{\Pr(Y_T = 0, Y_E = 1|X = d_k)\Pr(Y_T = 1, Y_E = 0|X = d_k)}, \qquad (5.14)$$

which quantifies the association between the toxicity and efficacy outcomes by parameter β_k. The probabilities $\Pr(Y_T = y_T, Y_E = y_E|X = d_k)$, $y_T, y_E \in \{0, 1\}$ can be obtained from β_k and the marginal probabilities $R(d_k)$ and $Q(d_k)$.

If the data for the first j included patients $\mathcal{D}_j = \{(x_l, y_{T,l}, y_{E,l}); l = 1, \ldots, j\}$ $(j = 1, \ldots, n_{\max})$ are obtained and j_k patients are treated at dose level k, the likelihood function is given by

$$\mathcal{L}(\mathcal{D}_j; \beta_k, R(d_k), Q(d_k))$$

$$= \prod_{k=1}^{K} \prod_{l=1}^{j_k} \prod_{y_T=0}^{1} \prod_{y_E=0}^{1} \{\Pr(Y_T = y_T, Y_E = y_E|X = d_k)\}^{I(Y_{T,kl}=y_T, Y_{E,kl}=y_E)}, (5.15)$$

where $I(\cdot)$ is the indicator function and $Y_{T,kl}$ and $Y_{E,kl}$ are the toxicity and efficacy outcomes, respectively, for the lth patient under dose level k among the first j included patients. It should be noted that, in the framework of this design, the probabilities of toxicity and efficacy associated with dose d_k, that is, $R(d_k)$ and $Q(d_k)$, are the parameters to be estimated. Yin et al. (2006) presented two different transformations to these probabilities for specification of the priors with or without incorporating the ordering constraint, and obtained the joint posterior distribution of the parameters. In addition, Yin et al. (2006) defined a set of admissible doses $\mathscr{D}_A$, which contains the doses satisfying the following two conditions:

$$\Pr(R(d_k) < \Gamma_T) > \xi_T \text{ and } \Pr(Q(d_k) > \Gamma_E) > \xi_E, \qquad (5.16)$$

where Γ_T and Γ_E are the prespecified maximum admissible toxicity and minimum admissible efficacy levels, respectively, and ξ_T and ξ_E are the corresponding pre-specified probability cutoffs. In addition, Yin et al. (2006) used the toxicity–efficacy odds-ratio contour. The OD is determined, such that the efficacy and toxicity probabilities $(Q(d_k), R(d_k))$ is located closest to the lower right corner $(1, 0)$. Those authors also considered a three-dimensional volume ratio through adding a third dimension of the conditional efficacy probability given the absence of toxicity. To calculate the odds ratio contour or volume, the posterior means were used.

The dose-finding algorithm of this approach is similar to that of the trade-off design proposed by Thall and Cook (2004) (see Sect. 5.4), as follows:

Step 1 Treat patients in the first cohort at the lowest dose level.

Step 2 Escalate the dose to the lowest untested dose level if the toxicity probability of the highest tested dose d^{last}, denoted by $R(d^{\text{last}})$, satisfies

$$\Pr(R(d^{\text{last}}) < \Gamma_T) > \xi_T^{\text{escl}} \qquad (5.17)$$

for some prespecified cutoff for dose escalation, $\xi_T^{\text{escl}} \geq \xi_T$.

Step 3 If a given dose level k satisfies Eq. (5.16), $d_k \in \mathscr{D}_A$. If Eq. (5.17) is not satisfied and $\mathscr{D}_A$ is an empty set (that is, $\mathscr{D}_A = \emptyset$), terminate the trial and do not select any dose, provided the minimum sample size is reached. Otherwise, allocate the most desirable dose from $\mathscr{D}_A$ as determined by the odds-ratio contour to patients in the next cohort, subject to the restriction that untested doses cannot be skipped during dose escalation or de-escalation.

Step 4 Once the maximum sample size $n_{\max}$ is reached, select the final dose in $\mathscr{D}_A$ that minimizes the toxicity–efficacy odds ratio.

Decisions on dose escalation, de-escalation, or maintenance should be based on data obtained for the tested doses. Thus, the dose must be escalated provided the highest attempted dose level has not exceeded the toxicity requirement in Eq. (5.17). If Eq. (5.17) is not satisfied, $\mathscr{D}_A = \emptyset$, and the minimum sample size is not reached, the most desirable dose as determined by the odds-ratio criterion, despite the fact that $\mathscr{D}_A = \emptyset$, is allocated to the next cohort of patients. In Yin et al. (2006), the minimum sample size is set to three.

5.3.5 Utility Design

Loke et al. (2006) proposed a phase I/II Bayesian utility design to incorporate both toxicity and efficacy in OD determination; this approach involves specification of a utility weight to quantify preferences regarding the consequences of possible actions. The design aims at making the optimal decision from among the set of possible actions, composed of dose escalation to the next highest dose level $\mathscr{A}_\uparrow$, dose de-escalation to the next lowest dose level $\mathscr{A}_\downarrow$, or maintenance of the same dose $\mathscr{A}_|$ after the data from each patient have been obtained. Suppose that some fixed set of doses are prespecified as $x \in \{d_1, \ldots, d_K\}$. Assuming independence between the toxicity and efficacy probabilities, the following four possible probabilities at each dose level k are given:

$$
\begin{aligned}
\beta_{1k} &= \Pr(Y_T = 0, Y_E = 0 | X = d_k) = \Pr(Y_T = 0 | X = d_k)\Pr(Y_E = 0 | X = d_k), \\
\beta_{2k} &= \Pr(Y_T = 0, Y_E = 1 | X = d_k) = \Pr(Y_T = 0 | X = d_k)\Pr(Y_E = 1 | X = d_k), \\
\beta_{3k} &= \Pr(Y_T = 1, Y_E = 0 | X = d_k) = \Pr(Y_T = 1 | X = d_k)\Pr(Y_E = 0 | X = d_k), \\
\beta_{4k} &= \Pr(Y_T = 1, Y_E = 1 | X = d_k) = \Pr(Y_T = 1 | X = d_k)\Pr(Y_E = 1 | X = d_k),
\end{aligned}
\tag{5.18}
$$

where $\boldsymbol{\beta} = (\beta_{1k}, \beta_{2k}, \beta_{3k}, \beta_{4k})$ is the parameter vector at each dose level k and is assumed to have a Dirichlet distribution. In addition, the multiple outcomes for Y_T and Y_E are assumed to have multinomial likelihood. Thus, the Bayesian conjugate analysis based on these assumptions yields a Dirichlet posterior distribution.

In this approach, utility values are assigned in order to weigh the consequences of each action of $\mathscr{A}_\uparrow$, $\mathscr{A}_|$, and $\mathscr{A}_\downarrow$, depending on the clinical importance of the combination of Y_T and Y_E and on some prespecified target probability of the combination associated with the OD.

The optimal action is the action that maximizes the expected utility on the posterior distribution, allowing for treatment of the next patient or cohort at the appropriate dose. Note that we classify this design as a rule-based design in that it does not allow for dependency or for strength borrowing among the dose levels. This design can also be adapted to handle scenarios in which the clinical investigators are interested in the toxicity alone.

5.4 Model-Based Designs

In model-based designs, a probability model denoted by π is assumed for the bivariate probability of both Y_T and Y_E with dose x of an agent:

$$
\Pr(Y_T = y_T, Y_E = y_E | X = x) = \pi_{y_T, y_E}(x, \boldsymbol{\beta}), \quad y_T, \ y_E \in \{0, 1\}, \tag{5.19}
$$

where $\boldsymbol{\beta}$ is a parameter vector. Because a phase I/II trial focuses on both toxicity and efficacy, a complex model is often used.

If the parameter estimation is based on the likelihood estimator, the number of parameters in the model is too large in the early stage of the trial for the parameters to be estimated; thus, an elaboration such as an initial dose escalation stage or a set of non-informative pseudo-data is required (see, e.g., O'Quigley et al. 2001). On the other hand, a Bayesian estimator allows for parameter estimation using the prior distribution. Thus, many of the model-based designs incorporating toxicity and efficacy are based on Bayesian approaches. The procedure employed for model-based designs based on Bayesian approaches is, in principle, identical to that of Chap. 3. That is, given the data for the first j included patients $\mathfrak{D}_j = \{(x_l, y_{T,l}, y_{E,l}); l = 1, \ldots, j\}$ ($j = 1, \ldots, n_{\max}$), the likelihood $\mathcal{L}(\mathfrak{D}_j; \boldsymbol{\beta})$ is obtained according to the forms of the assumed model. Then, the prior distribution of $\boldsymbol{\beta}$ is updated to the posterior. To avoid the risk of treating patients at a dose with either inadmissibly high toxicity or inadmissibly low efficacy, in the Bayesian framework, the OD may be defined as the dose maximizing the posterior probability of success, $\Pr(\pi_{0,1}(x, \boldsymbol{\beta}) \geq \Gamma_E)$. In addition, this dose may be required to satisfy

$$\Pr(\pi_T(x, \boldsymbol{\beta}) \leq \Gamma_T | \mathfrak{D}_j) \geq \xi_T \tag{5.20}$$

and

$$\Pr(\pi_E(x, \boldsymbol{\beta}) \geq \Gamma_E | \mathfrak{D}_j) \geq \xi_E \tag{5.21}$$

or

$$\Pr(\pi_{0,1}(x, \boldsymbol{\beta}) \geq \Gamma_E | \mathfrak{D}_j) \geq \xi_E, \tag{5.22}$$

where Γ_T and Γ_E are the prespecified maximum admissible toxicity and minimum admissible efficacy levels, respectively; ξ_T and ξ_E are the corresponding prespecified probability cutoffs; and $\pi_T(x, \boldsymbol{\beta}) = \pi_{1,0}(x, \boldsymbol{\beta}) + \pi_{1,1}(x, \boldsymbol{\beta})$ and $\pi_E(x, \boldsymbol{\beta}) = \pi_{0,1}(x, \boldsymbol{\beta}) + \pi_{1,1}(x, \boldsymbol{\beta})$.

5.4.1 Trinomial-Ordinal-Outcome Design

Thall and Russell (1998) proposed a phase I/II trial design in which the patients' toxicity and efficacy outcomes, Y_T and Y_E, are captured by a trinomial-ordinal outcome U, that is, $\{U = 0\} = \{Y_T = 0, Y_E = 0\}$, $\{U = 1\} = \{Y_T = 0, Y_E = 1\}$, and $\{U = 2\} = \{Y_T = 1\}$. Then, Eq. (5.19) can be rewritten as

$$\Pr(U = u | X = x) = \pi_u(x, \boldsymbol{\beta}), \ u \in \{0, 1, 2\}. \tag{5.23}$$

Thall and Russell (1998) assumed the following proportional odds model for the trinomial-ordinal outcome because, in general, the probability of $U = 0$, denoted by $\pi_0(x, \boldsymbol{\beta})$ and the probability of $U = 2$, denoted by $\pi_2(x, \boldsymbol{\beta})$, are assumed to be decreasing and increasing functions of dose x, respectively:

$$\log \frac{\pi_1(x, \boldsymbol{\beta}) + \pi_2(x, \boldsymbol{\beta})}{1 - \{\pi_1(x, \boldsymbol{\beta}) + \pi_2(x, \boldsymbol{\beta})\}} = \beta_1 + \beta_3 x,$$

$$\log \frac{\pi_2(x, \boldsymbol{\beta})}{1 - \pi_2(x, \boldsymbol{\beta})} = \beta_2 + \beta_3 x, \tag{5.24}$$

where $\boldsymbol{\beta} = (\beta_1, \beta_2, \beta_3)$, $\beta_1 > \beta_2$, and $\beta_3 > 0$ to ensure the monotonic relationships of $\pi_0(x, \boldsymbol{\beta})$ and $\pi_2(x, \boldsymbol{\beta})$ with dose x. In this model, the dose effect is the same across the cumulative logits. The assumption of proportionality can be relaxed by assuming different slope parameters for β_3. The parameters are estimated via Bayesian inference. The prior for each parameter of $\boldsymbol{\beta}$ is assumed to be independently uniform over some range prespecified through discussion with clinical investigators.

This design considers a dose to be admissible if both $\Pr(\pi_2(x, \boldsymbol{\beta}) \leq \Gamma_T) \geq \xi_T$ and $\Pr(\pi_1(x, \boldsymbol{\beta}) \geq \Gamma_E) \geq \xi_E$ are satisfied, and inadmissible otherwise (see Eqs. 5.20 and 5.22). Therefore, such an admissible dose is used to treat each enrolled patient during a course of the trial and is identified as the OD at the end of the trial. If there exists no such admissible dose, the trial is terminated. As suggested by Thall and Cheng (1999), if $\Pr(\pi_1(x, \boldsymbol{\beta}) \geq \Gamma_E)$ is very close to the largest value for several doses, the definition of the OD can be modified to the dose among these candidate doses that maximizes $\Pr(\pi_1(x, \boldsymbol{\beta}) \leq \Gamma_E)$.

There is one major difficulty associated with this design: in cases where all doses have admissible toxicity, but higher doses show higher efficacy, the employed dose is not escalated to the more effective doses with high probability. Thus, the design may fail to find the OD among several admissible doses. Other difficulties are that the proportional odds model, although parsimonious, may be too restrictive in some situations, and that the design cannot directly investigate the relationship between dose and each response with regard to toxicity and efficacy, because the toxicity and efficacy outcomes are reduced to a trinomial-ordinal outcome in the proportional odds model.

Zhang et al. (2006) presented a simple modified version of the design proposed by Thall and Russell (1998). They called this design "TriCRM," because it generalizes the continual reassessment method (CRM) (see Sects. 3.2 and 3.3) in that the patient toxicity and efficacy outcomes are considered as a trinomial-ordinal outcome. Those authors assumed the following continuation-ratio model for the above trinomial-ordinal outcome:

$$\log \left\{ \frac{\pi_1(x, \boldsymbol{\beta})}{\pi_0(x, \boldsymbol{\beta})} \right\} = \beta_1 + \beta_3 x,$$

$$\log \frac{\pi_2(x, \boldsymbol{\beta})}{1 - \pi_2(x, \boldsymbol{\beta})} = \beta_2 + \beta_4 x, \tag{5.25}$$

where $\boldsymbol{\beta} = (\beta_1, \beta_2, \beta_3, \beta_4)$, $\beta_1 > \beta_2$, and $\beta_3, \beta_4 > 0$. This model does not employ the proportional odds assumption. The two following functions are used for dose assignment:

$$\delta_1(x, \boldsymbol{\beta}) = I\{\pi_2(x, \boldsymbol{\beta}) < \Gamma_T\}, \tag{5.26}$$

$$\delta_2(x, \boldsymbol{\beta}) = \pi_1(x, \boldsymbol{\beta}) - w\pi_2(x, \boldsymbol{\beta}), \tag{5.27}$$

where I is an indicator function and $0 \leq w \leq 1$ is the weight for $\pi_2(x, \boldsymbol{\beta})$. For a given estimate of $\boldsymbol{\beta}$, Eq. (5.26) is first used to choose the admissible dose set, denoted by $\mathscr{D}_A$, from the set of prespecified doses, denoted by $\mathscr{D} = \{d_1, \ldots, d_K\}$. Equation (5.27), which represents the difference between the success probability and toxicity probability if $w = 1$ and the success probability if $w = 0$, is then used to find the dose maximizing the value of $\delta_2(x, \boldsymbol{\beta})$. This dose is used to treat each enrolled patient or cohort during a course of the trial and is identified as the OD at the end of the trial.

5.4.2 Efficacy–Toxicity Trade-off Design

Thall and Cook (2004) proposed a phase I/II design to solve the difficulties associated with the design of Thall and Russell (1998). For the above trinomial ordinal outcome, those authors assumed a continuation-ratio model. They further formulated the bivariate probability of the binary toxicity and efficacy outcomes in terms of the marginal toxicity probability $\pi_T(x, \boldsymbol{\beta})$, efficacy probability $\pi_E(x, \boldsymbol{\beta})$, and an association parameter ρ. Specifically, in this approach, $\pi_T(x, \boldsymbol{\beta})$ and $\pi_E(x, \boldsymbol{\beta})$ are given by

$$\pi_T(x, \boldsymbol{\beta}) = \pi_{1,0}(x, \boldsymbol{\beta}) + \pi_{1,1}(x, \boldsymbol{\beta}) = \text{logit}^{-1}\{\eta_T(x, \boldsymbol{\beta})\}) \tag{5.28}$$

and

$$\pi_E(x, \boldsymbol{\beta}) = \pi_{0,1}(x, \boldsymbol{\beta}) + \pi_{1,1}(x, \boldsymbol{\beta}) = \text{logit}^{-1}\{\eta_E(x, \boldsymbol{\beta})\}), \tag{5.29}$$

where $\eta_T(x, \boldsymbol{\beta}) = \beta_1 + \beta_2 x$ and $\eta_E(x, \boldsymbol{\beta}) = \beta_3 + \beta_4 x + \beta_5 x^2$. Therefore, the model has a vector of six parameters, $\boldsymbol{\beta} = (\beta_1, \beta_2, \beta_3, \beta_4, \beta_5, \rho)$. It should be noted that the toxicity is assumed to be monotonic in x, but the efficacy is assumed to be quadratically non-monotonic in x. The latter model allows the design to be used for trials of targeted agents, for which $\pi_E(x, \boldsymbol{\beta})$ may increase for lower doses and then reach a plateau, or possibly decrease for higher doses. To consider the association between the binary toxicity and efficacy outcomes, the following Gumbel model (Murtaugh and Fisher 1990), also called the Morgenstern distribution (suppressing x and $\boldsymbol{\beta}$), is used:

$$\pi_{y_T, y_E} = \pi_T^{y_T}(1 - \pi_T)^{1-y_T}\pi_E^{y_E}(1 - \pi_E)^{1-y_E}$$
$$+ (-1)^{y_T+y_E}\pi_T(1 - \pi_T)\pi_E(1 - \pi_E)\frac{\exp(\rho) - 1}{\exp(\rho) + 1}. \tag{5.30}$$

Thall and Cook (2004) used a set of efficacy–toxicity trade-off contours that partition the two-dimensional domain of the possible values of outcome probabilities (π_E, π_T) to treat successive patient cohorts at admissible doses and to find the OD, instead of directly using Eqs. (5.20) and (5.21).

5.4.3 Repeated Sequential Probability Ratio Test Designs

O'Quigley et al. (2001) proposed phase I/II designs applicable to HIV dose-finding studies. To determine the OD that maximizes $\Pr(Y_T = 0, Y_E = 1 | X = x)$ over dose $x \in \{d_1, \ldots, d_K\}$, O'Quigley et al. (2001) considered the dose–toxicity curve $R(x) = \Pr(Y_T = 1 | X = x)$, dose–efficacy curve $Q'(x) = \Pr(Y_E = 1 | Y_T = 0, X = x)$, and dose–success curve $P(x) = Q'(x)\{1 - R(x)\}$. Specifically, they defined the dose level k^* such that $P(d_{k^*}) > P(d_k)$ for all k not equal to $k^*(\in \{1, \ldots, K\})$ as the OD. This dose is called the "MSD," as defined by Zohar and O'Quigley (2006a), and this concept was extended to the "safe MSD" by Zohar and O'Quigley (2006b), i.e., the MSD satisfying the safety restriction. Zohar and O'Quigley (2006b) investigated the optimal design for estimating the MSD in phase I/II trials evaluating both toxicity and efficacy based on the concepts of O'Quigley et al. (2002), and gave examples of comparisons between the optimal design and the designs of O'Quigley et al. (2001), Braun (2002), Ivanova (2003), and Thall and Cook (2004) in various scenarios.

For estimation of the above three curves, they presented three approaches based on empirical estimates without relying on any structure, under-parameterized models imposing any structure, and compromise structure lying between these two. Here, we outline the third approach. First, O'Quigley et al. (2001) used the likelihood version of the CRM (see O'Quigley and Shen 1996 and Sect. 3.2.2.2) to target a certain low-toxicity probability level. Second, in conjunction with accumulation of information at tested levels yielding success, the design proposed by O'Quigley et al. (2001) uses the repeated sequential probability ratio test (SPRT) at increasing dose levels, as follows: letting $\Gamma_{E,0}^*$ and $\Gamma_{E,1}^* (> \Gamma_{E,0}^*)$ denote the values for the probability of success that are regarded to be unsatisfactory and satisfactory, respectively, at dose d_k, hypothesis testing of $H_0 : P(d_k) = \Gamma_{E,0}^*$ versus $H_1 : P(d_k) = \Gamma_{E,1}^*$ is performed. The type-I and -II errors are, respectively, fixed at $\alpha = \Pr(H_1 | H_0)$ and $\beta = \Pr(H_0 | H_1)$. After enrollment of the first j patients, the following are calculated:

$$s_j(d_k) = \log \frac{\Gamma_{E,0}^*(1 - \Gamma_{E,1}^*)}{\Gamma_{E,1}^*(1 - \Gamma_{E,0}^*)} \tag{5.31}$$

$$\times \left[\sum_{l \leq j} y_{E,l} I(x_l = d_k, y_{T,l} = 0) - j \left\{ \log \frac{\Gamma_{E,0}^*}{\Gamma_{E,1}^*} - \log \frac{\Gamma_{E,0}^*(1 - \Gamma_{E,1}^*)}{\Gamma_{E,1}^*(1 - \Gamma_{E,0}^*)} \right\} \right],$$

where x_l, $y_{T,l}$, and $y_{T,l}$ are the dose, observed toxicity outcome, and observed efficacy outcome for the lth patient for $l = 1, \ldots, j$, respectively. The SPRT determines that the trial is continued provided

$$\log\left(\frac{1-\beta}{\alpha}\right) < s_j(d_k) < \log\left(\frac{\beta}{1-\alpha}\right). \tag{5.32}$$

In practice, if for the jth included patient, $s_j(d_k) > \log\{\beta/(1-\alpha)\}$, H_1 is accepted and the agent is determined to be promising at d_k. If $s_j(d_k) < \log\{(1-\beta)/\alpha\}$, H_0 is accepted and the agent is not sufficiently effective at d_k, yielding removal of d_k and lower doses. The target toxicity probability level is increased to $\Gamma_T + \delta$ until its prespecified maximum toxicity probability level, where δ is a prespecified increment and may equal zero; then, the trial continues at d_{k+1}.

5.4.4 Utility Design

Wang and Day (2010) proposed a phase I/II design based on the Bayesian expected utility. The proposed design assumes a joint model for thresholds for doses producing toxicity and efficacy responses. In that approach, it is assumed that the toxicity or efficacy outcome, i.e., Y_T or Y_E, occurs if the dose $x(\in \{d_1 \ldots, d_K\})$ exceeds the patient's threshold dose for that outcome, ξ_T or ξ_E. Therefore, one of the following four joint outcomes will occur: if and only if $\xi_T > x$ and $\xi_E > x$, $Y_T = 0$ and $Y_E = 0$; if and only if $\xi_T > x$ and $\xi_E \le x$, $Y_T = 0$ and $Y_E = 1$; if and only if $\xi_T \le x$ and $\xi_E > x$, $Y_T = 1$ and $Y_E = 0$; and if and only if $\xi_T \le x$ and $\xi_E \le x$, $Y_T = 1$ and $Y_E = 1$. The probabilities of the four joint outcomes are represented using joint density of the thresholds $p(\xi_T, \xi_E)$:

$$\Pr(Y_T = 0, Y_E = 0 | X = x) = \int_x^\infty \int_x^\infty p(\xi_T, \xi_E) d\xi_T d\xi_E, \tag{5.33}$$

$$\Pr(Y_T = 0, Y_E = 1 | X = x) = \int_x^\infty \int_0^x p(\xi_T, \xi_E) d\xi_T d\xi_E, \tag{5.34}$$

$$\Pr(Y_T = 1, Y_E = 0 | X = x) = \int_0^x \int_x^\infty p(\xi_T, \xi_E) d\xi_T d\xi_E, \tag{5.35}$$

$$\Pr(Y_T = 1, Y_E = 1 | X = x) = \int_0^x \int_0^x p(\xi_T, \xi_E) d\xi_T d\xi_E. \tag{5.36}$$

The individual thresholds for toxicity and efficacy are assumed to jointly have a bivariate log-normal distribution with mean vector μ and variance–covariance matrix Σ, where

$$\mu = \begin{pmatrix} \mu_T \\ \mu_E \end{pmatrix} \text{ and } \Sigma = \begin{pmatrix} \sigma_T^2 & \sigma_T\sigma_E\rho \\ \sigma_T\sigma_E\rho & \sigma_E^2 \end{pmatrix}. \tag{5.37}$$

Thus, the parameter to be estimated is $\boldsymbol{\beta} = (\mu_T, \mu_E, \sigma_T, \sigma_E, \rho)$. Parameter estimation can be conducted via Bayesian inference. Let U_{y_T, y_E} denote the utility given to the toxicity and efficacy outcomes. Given the data $\mathfrak{D}_j$ for the jth patient, the Bayesian expected utility for the next patient or cohort is given as a function of dose by $\sum_{y_T \in \{0,1\}} \sum_{y_E \in \{0,1\}} U_{y_T, y_E} E_{\boldsymbol{\beta}} \{\Pr(Y_T = y_T, Y_E = y_E) | \mathfrak{D}_j\}$, where $E_{\boldsymbol{\beta}}$ is a posterior expectation. The dose that maximizes this expected utility can be regarded as the OD.

5.4.5 Other Designs

Whitehead et al. (2004, 2006a, b) assumed two logistic models as parsimonious models, for the toxicity probability and the conditional efficacy probability given the absence of toxicity, respectively:

$$\pi_T(x, \boldsymbol{\beta}) = \frac{\exp(\beta_1 + \beta_2 \log x)}{1 + \exp(\beta_1 + \beta_2 \log x)} \tag{5.38}$$

and

$$\pi_{E|T}(x, \boldsymbol{\beta}) = \frac{\exp(\beta_3 + \beta_4 \log x)}{1 + \exp(\beta_3 + \beta_4 \log x)}, \tag{5.39}$$

where $\boldsymbol{\beta} = (\beta_1, \beta_2, \beta_3, \beta_4)$. In this approach, the parameters are estimated using the Bayesian inference, where the prior specification is based on the pseudo-data and mode estimates, because of the conformity of the Bayesian inference to the likelihood inference, and because this allows for fitting on commonly used frequentist software for logistic regression. The dose is recommended through making the decision that maximizes the value of the "patient gain" or "variance gain" (see Whitehead and Brunier (1995) and Sect. 3.4), provided the safety restrictions are taken as an option. To treat the next enrolled patient or cohort, the former chooses the dose that maximizes the product of Eqs. (5.38) and (5.39), that is, $\Pr(Y_T = 0, Y_E = 1)$, whereas the latter selects the dose that enables us to accurately estimate the limits of the therapeutic window.

It should be noted that the toxicity and efficacy considered here are intended to pertain to not only oncological topics but also other therapeutic fields; thus, they are defined differently than the standard definitions, as a dose-limiting event (DLE) and a desirable outcome (DO), respectively. Occurrence of a DLE will generate concern among the clinical investigators or independent data monitoring committee responsible for the trial conduct, indicating that progression to a higher dose may be unwise. Therefore, this definition includes the concept of DLT in some sense. The DO may be a beneficial therapeutic effect, a surrogate eventually resulting in benefit in patients, or a biomarker believed to reflect the intended mechanisms of action of an agent in healthy volunteers.

5.5 Model-Assisted Designs

5.5.1 Toxicity and Efficacy Probability Interval (TEPI) Design

Li et al. (2016) developed a toxicity and efficacy probability interval (TEPI) design in adoptive cell therapy. The TEPI design is a natural extension of the modified toxicity probability interval (mTPI) design (Ji et al. 2010) (see Sect. 4.2) that considers the joint unit probability mass (JUPM) for the toxicity and efficacy probability intervals. Thus, this design is also simple and transparent, because all decision rules, i.e., dose escalation, de-escalation, and maintenance rules, can be provided prior to trial initiation.

Let $\pi_{T,k}$ ($k = 1, \ldots, K$) denote the toxicity probability that increases with dose level k and let $\pi_{E,k}$ indicate the efficacy probability. The latter may increase initially before reaching a plateau such that minimal improvement or even decreasing efficacy may be observed with increasing dose. It is assumed that $\pi_{T,k}$ has an independent beta distribution denoted by $\text{Beta}(a_T, b_T)$, and that $\pi_{E,k}$ has an independent beta distribution denoted by $\text{Beta}(a_E, b_E)$.

Considering the two-dimensional unit square $(0, 1) \times (0, 1)$ in the real space, the JUPM for each interval combination $(a, b) \times (c, d)$ is defined by

$$\text{JUPM}_{(a,b)}^{(c,d)} = \frac{\Pr\left\{\pi_{T,k} \in (a, b), \pi_{E,k} \in (c, d)\right\}}{(b - a)(d - c)}, \ 0 < a < b < 1, \ 0 < c < d < 1,$$

(5.40)

where the numerator $\Pr\left\{\pi_{T,k} \in (a, b), \pi_{E,k} \in (c, d)\right\}$ incorporates the posterior probabilities π_T and π_E falling in the (a, b) and (c, d) intervals, respectively, given the administered dose level and the corresponding observed toxicity and efficacy data. The "winning" interval combination that achieves the maximum JUPM among all interval combinations is identified, and the corresponding decision (escalation, de-escalation, or maintenance of the current dose) for that combination is selected for treatment of the next cohort of patients.

5.5.2 Bayesian Optimal Interval Design Considering Both Toxicity and Efficacy (BOIN-ET Design)

Takeda et al. (2018) extended the Bayesian optimal interval (BOIN) design of Liu and Yuan (2015) (see Sect. 4.4) to a design that identifies an OD considering both efficacy and toxicity, called the "BOIN-ET" design.

Let $\pi_{T,k}$ and $\pi_{E,k}$ denote the toxicity probability and efficacy probability at dose level k, respectively, for $k = 1, \ldots, K$. In addition, let Γ_T and Γ_E denote the target toxicity probability level and efficacy probability level, respectively.

In the BOIN-ET design, six point hypotheses are formulated for $\pi_{T,k}$ and $\pi_{E,k}$ as follows:

$$
\begin{aligned}
H_{1,k} &: \pi_{T,k} = \Gamma_{T,1}, \ \pi_{E,k} = \Gamma_{E,1}, \\
H_{2,k} &: \pi_{T,k} = \Gamma_{T,1}, \ \pi_{E,k} = \Gamma_{E}, \\
H_{3,k} &: \pi_{T,k} = \Gamma_{T}, \ \pi_{E,k} = \Gamma_{E,1}, \\
H_{4,k} &: \pi_{T,k} = \Gamma_{T}, \ \pi_{E,k} = \Gamma_{E}, \\
H_{5,k} &: \pi_{T,k} = \Gamma_{T,2}, \ \pi_{E,k} = \Gamma_{E,1}, \\
H_{6,k} &: \pi_{T,k} = \Gamma_{T,2}, \ \pi_{E,k} = \Gamma_{E}, \quad (5.41)
\end{aligned}
$$

where $\Gamma_{T,1}$ denotes the highest toxicity probability regarded to be below the MTD, $\Gamma_{T,2}$ denotes the lowest toxicity probability regarded to be above the MTD, and $\Gamma_{E,1}$ denotes the highest efficacy probability regarded to be sub-therapeutic such that another dose level should be explored. $\Gamma_{E} - \Gamma_{E,1}$ corresponds to the effect size or minimal difference of practical interest to be discerned from the target efficacy probability Γ_{E}. When each hypothesis is true, correct and incorrect decisions are given. The cutoff values required for the dose allocation to be compared with the estimated toxicity and efficacy probabilities are calculated by minimizing the posterior probability of incorrect decisions. Consequently, similar to the BOIN design, a dose-finding algorithm is obtained.

The BOIN-ET design is also simple and transparent, because all decision rules can be prespecified prior to trial initiation.

5.6 Overview of Other Designs and Discussion of Related Topics

5.6.1 Designs for Molecularly Targeted Agents

Targeted therapies in oncology use agents or other substances such as small molecules, monoclonal antibodies, dendritic cells, and labeled radionuclides to attack specific disease cells while sparing normal cells. These targeted therapies have mechanisms of action based on drug-receptor (target) theory. That is, if an agent or substance with an OD can be delivered to the target, its efficacy manifests as complete termination of disease cells or their growth, without causing damage to normal cells (i.e., in the form of toxicity) (see Le Tourneau et al. 2010). Therefore, theoretically or ideally, compared with CAs, targeted therapeutic agents are presupposed to have less toxicity and nonmonotonically increasing efficacy with increasing dose. Further, either the dose–toxicity or dose–efficacy relationships may have an umbrella shape (Conolly and Lutz 2004; Lagarde et al. 2015) or a plateau shape (Morgan et al. 2003; Postel-Vinay et al. 2011; Robert et al. 2014; Paoletti et al. 2014). Hence, the highest efficacy is achieved at the dose below the MTD. See also, Chaps. 3 and 4 of the book by Hirakawa et al. (2018).

There exist some phase I/II trial designs that loosen the assumption of monotonicity in the dose–efficacy relationship (see, e.g., Hunsberger et al. 2005, Polley and Cheung 2008, Hoering et al. 2013, Yin et al. 2013, Cai et al. 2014, Zang et al. 2014, Wages and Tait 2015, Riviere et al. 2018, Mozgunov and Jaki 2019 and Muenz et al. 2019 for a binary efficacy outcome, and Hirakawa 2012 and Yeung et al. 2015, 2017 for a continuous efficacy outcome). In particular, software to implement the design of Zang et al. (2014) is available as Shiny online applications from http://www.trialdesign.org/.

5.6.2 Designs for Binary Toxicity and Continuous Efficacy Outcomes

Bekele and Shen (2005) presented a dose-finding design for cases in which toxicity is considered to be a binary outcome. In that approach, however, the efficacy is considered to be a continuous outcome through expression of a biomarker. A probit model with a latent variable is given for the relationship between dose and toxicity, and a model that considers toxicity and efficacy is established based on a state-space model for the relationship between dose and biomarker expression.

Hirakawa (2012) proposed a dose-finding method for analysis of correlating bivariate binary toxicity and continuous efficacy outcomes by means of the factorization models in single-agent and two-agent combination trials. Ezzalfani et al. (2019) proposed a design to identify the optimal dose through using joint modeling of repeated binary toxicity and continuous efficacy outcomes from the first two cycles.

5.6.3 Designs for Ordinal Toxicity and Efficacy Outcomes

Houede et al. (2010) proposed a design that searches for clinically appropriate combinations of doses of both drugs in a combination therapy featuring a chemical preparation and a biological preparation, with respect to the ordinal categorical responses of toxicity and efficacy. Some of the features of this method are that the marginal probabilities of toxicity and efficacy are given as functions of the dose combination, using an extension of the model developed by Aranda-Ordaz (1981); that the relationship between the toxicity probability and the efficacy probability is given using the Gaussian copula; that the dose combination is assigned by optimizing the posterior expected utility of the patient outcome; and that the case in which the toxicity is excessively high and an efficacy evaluation cannot be performed is considered.

5.6.4 Designs for Time-to-Toxicity and Time-to-Efficacy Outcomes

Yuan and Yin (2009) proposed a design considering the time until the advent of toxicity or efficacy. They postulated a proportional hazards model (Cox 1972) and a cure rate model (Berkson and Gage 1952) for the time until toxicity and efficacy are observed, respectively. In particular, the latter model openly postulates that a certain patient fraction is resistant to treatment (thus, those patients are not cured). In this design, dose finding is performed based on the trade-off between toxicity and efficacy using the ratio between the area under the curve (AUC) for toxicity and the AUC for efficacy.

Liu and Johnson (2016) developed a Bayesian phase I/II dose-finding trial design that considers toxicity and efficacy outcomes, where these outcomes are modeled using a Bayesian dynamic model with no stringent parametric assumptions on the shapes of the dose–toxicity and dose–efficacy curves. In addition, those researchers extended the proposed design for delayed outcomes. Readers can obtain the program used to simulate this design at http://www.stat.tamu.edu/~vjohnson/.

5.6.5 Designs for Finding Maximum Tolerated Dose and Schedule

Li et al. (2008) focused on the constraint of matrix ordering in that, in a matrix having a toxicity probability corresponding to each dose and schedule level combination, an ordinal relationship exists when focus is placed on either dose or schedule. (For example, when focus is placed on dose (or schedule), the toxicity probability increases with increases in that level.) However, there is no ordering constraint in terms of the efficacy probability. Li et al. (2008) presented a design that achieved this constraint through isotonic transformation, and found the maximum tolerated dose and schedule with the lowest toxicity but highest efficacy by assuming a global cross-ratio model for the simultaneous toxicity and efficacy probabilities as binary responses. In addition, they presented a design called "CRM+AR." In the first stage of CRM+AR, the MTD is identified by applying the CRM (see Sects. 3.2 and 3.3) to each schedule. In the second stage, assignment of the dose and schedule combination is performed using adaptive randomization (AR) via the posterior probabilities that the toxicity probability does not exceed the target toxicity probability level and that the efficacy probability is at the target efficacy probability level at least.

Guo et al. (2016) proposed a phase I/II design to find the optimal dose-schedule combination, through using a Bayesian dynamic model for the joint effects of dose and schedule.

5.6.6 Designs for Drug Combinations

Huang et al. (2007) proposed a dose-finding design for phase I/II trials in which a phase I trial focusing on toxicity evaluation in combination therapy involving two drugs or treatments is conducted in parallel with a phase II trial focusing on evaluation of the resulting therapeutic effect. This design involves the following steps:

Step 1   The two-dimensional plane configured from the doses of the two drugs is divided into multiple zones (these zones include combinations of doses for each drug, and each combination of doses in the same zone is randomly allocated to the patients using a permuted block method). A modified 3 + 3 design (Storer 1989) (see Sect. 2.2) is applied for dose escalation by regarding each zone itself as a dose level. This allows identification of the zones with tolerable toxicity (the escalation phase).

Step 2   By comparing the response rates, which are evaluated in terms of the efficacy of the dose combinations contained in the identified tolerable zones (the arms in the phase II trial arm, so to speak), with the response rate of the initial zone (i.e., the lowest combination level) on the posterior distribution, patients are treated according to the arm with the highest efficacy via adaptive randomization.

After initiation of adaptive randomization in Step 2, the toxicity is evaluated together with the efficacy. As a result, assignment of arms with a high toxicity probability and a low efficacy probability is terminated. If the assignment probability of an arm is low according to the adaptive randomization, assignment of that arm is suspended. Huang et al. (2007) provided an application example involving investigation of simultaneous and sequential combination therapies involving administration of low-dose decitabine and Ara-C to relapsed/refractory acute myeloid leukemia patients.

Whitehead et al. (2011) generalized the Bayesian phase I dose escalation design for binary toxicity of a single agent described by Whitehead et al. (2010) into a phase I/II design for determining the binary toxicity and efficacy of a combination of two drugs. This design is based on assumption of monotonicity in the relationship between the relative strength of the dose combination and the multinomial distribution of the bivariate toxicity and efficacy outcome. The prior is based on a flat prior in which each multinomial distribution has the same probability, or an informative prior in which pseudo-data is used. Because the multinomial model is assumed for each dose combination and does not accommodate dependency among the combinations, this design may be regarded as a rule-based design.

Hirakawa (2012) presented a dose-finding design for a single drug and a combination therapy of two drugs, in which the toxicity and efficacy are correlated and observed as a binary and a continuous quantity, respectively. The author conducted simulations to compare the proposed design with that of Bekele and Shen (2005), showing that the former had superior operating characteristics to the latter.

Mandrekar et al. (2007) provided a generalization of the TriCRM design to find the OD for two-agent combination. Furthermore, Mandrekar and colleagues (2010) gave a review of designs based on proportional odds and continuation-ratio models to find the OD of a single-agent or a two-agent combination.

Riviere et al. (2015) proposed a design for trials combining a cytotoxic agent with an MTA. In this approach, the toxicity is modeled using a logistic regression model and the efficacy is modeled using a novel proportional hazard model, which accounts for the plateau in the MTA dose–efficacy curve.

5.6.7 Designs for Covariate Information

Thall et al. (2008) proposed a dose-finding design individualized for each patient as an extension of the design of Thall and Cook (2004). This design utilizes covariate information for patients, similar to the design of Babb and Rogatko (2001). Note that, instead of application of the Gumbel model to the relationship between the toxicity probability and efficacy probability, a more generalized Gaussian copula was considered based on the dependence between the random variables.

Guo and Yuan (2017) proposed a design to find the optimal dose for treating patients with a molecularly targeted agent, according to patient's biomarker status. This design models the ordinal toxicity and efficacy using the latent-variable approach, and uses canonical partial least squares to extract a small number of components to be included as covariates.

Kakurai et al. (2019) developed a method for the optimal dose individualization and covariate selection that is associated with efficacy and toxicity, through using Bayesian least absolute shrinkage and selection operator.

5.6.8 Designs for Toxicity and Other Outcomes

Thall et al. (2001) extended the CRM by incorporating the perspective of feasibility. This approach was adopted to address the situations arising in dendritic-cell activated T-cell injection trials, in which the injection target number of T-cells cannot necessarily be obtained through ex vivo culturing. In this design, the feasibility is defined as the posterior probability of whether the probability of T-cell infusibility is less than the target probability. In addition, for immunotherapy trials of patients exhibiting relapse of a hematologic malignancy after an allogeneic bone marrow transplant, Thall et al. (2002) proposed a design that searches for the injection timing for allogeneic donor lymphocytes and the appropriate mylotarg dose based on the patient data on toxicity, the time until recovery of the absolute neutrophil count, and the survival time.

Braun (2002) proposed a bivariate CRM (bCRM) that, based on the CRM working model, simultaneously considers the two variables of toxicity and another competing response. This design can also describe the relationship between the dose and each of those responses. Here, the pair of random variables representing the toxicity response and another competing response for treatment of a patient at dose x is denoted (Y, Z) (where the observed value $y = 1$ if there is toxicity and $y = 0$ otherwise, and $z = 1$ if the other competing response is present and $z = 0$ otherwise). The correlation parameter between those responses is represented by ρ ($0 < \rho < 1$). Then, in the bCRM, the bivariate distribution of (Y, Z) for dose x is given by

$$
\begin{aligned}
f(y, z|x) = {} & C(\psi_1(x, \beta_1), \psi_2(x, \beta_2), r) \\
& \times \{\psi_1(x, \beta_1)\}^y \{1 - \psi_1(x, \beta_1)\}^{(1-y)} \{\psi_2(x, \beta_2)\}^z \{1 - \psi_2(x, \beta_2)\}^{(1-z)} \\
& \times r^{yz}(1 - r)^{(1-yz)},
\end{aligned}
\tag{5.42}
$$

where $C(\cdot)$ is a normalizing constant, $\psi_1(x, \beta_1)$ is the working model for toxicity with one parameter β_1, and $\psi_2(x, \beta_2)$ is the working model for the other competing response with one parameter β_2. The possible ranges for parameters β_1 and β_2 differ depending on the form of the working model, but in the case of power models and logistic models with these parameters as slopes, $\beta_1 > 0$ and $\beta_2 > 0$. In addition, the non-informative prior distribution with respect to the parameters of interest (β_1, β_2, ρ) is assumed to be

$$
g(\beta_1, \beta_2, \rho) = 6\rho(1 - \rho)\exp\{-(\beta_1 + \beta_2)\}.
\tag{5.43}
$$

By combining the likelihood obtained from Eq. (5.42) with the prior distribution given in Eq. (5.43), and by obtaining a posterior distribution for the parameters in accordance with Bayes' theorem, it is possible to calculate their posterior means. Estimates of the toxicity probability and the probability of the other competing response can be obtained by substituting the posterior mean for β_1 into the working model for toxicity and the posterior mean for β_2 into the working model for the competing response. The dose that should be used to treat the next enrolled patient is determined as the dose that minimizes the Euclidean distance between these estimates and the target toxicity and competing response probability levels.

Note that Ivanova et al. (2009) proposed a design considering proof-of-concept trials, dose-response trials, and dose-ranging trials. Further, O'Quigley et al. (2010) discussed an algorithm for dose finding using the pharmacokinetic response as the target, focusing on bridging trials.

5.6.9 Decision-Theoretic and Optimal Designs

Zhou et al. (2006) presented a design based on Bayesian decision theory in which the efficacy is taken to be a continuous quantity; this approach is based on Whitehead et al. (2001), Patterson et al. (1999), and Whitehead et al. (2006b). In addition, Fan and Wang (2006) presented a dose-finding design based on a decision theory that considers the bandit problem, as in Leung and Wang (2002). A design based on D-optimal design criteria (Dragalin and Fedorov 2006; Fedorov and Wu 2007; Dragalin et al. 2008; Padmanabhan et al. 2010; and Pronzato 2010) has also been proposed.

References

Aranda-Ordaz, F.J.: On two families of transformations to additivity for binary response data. Biometrika **68**(2), 357–363 (1981)

Babb, J.S., Rogatko, A.: Patient specific dosing in a cancer phase I clinical trial. Stat. Med. **20**(14), 2079–2090 (2001)

Bekele, B.N., Shen, Y.: A Bayesian approach to jointly modeling toxicity and biomarker expression in a phase I/II dose-finding trial. Biometrics **61**(2), 344–354 (2005)

Berkson, J., Gage, R.P.: Survival curve for cancer patients following treatment. J. Am. Stat. Assoc. **47**(259), 501–515 (1952)

Braun, T.M.: The bivariate continual reassessment method: extending the CRM to phase I trials of two competing outcomes. Control. Clin. Trials **23**(3), 240–256 (2002)

Cai, C., Yuan, Y., Ji, Y.: A Bayesian dose finding design for oncology clinical trials of combinational biological agents. J. Roy. Stat. Soc. Ser. C Appl. Stat. **63**(1), 159–173 (2014)

Conolly, R.B., Lutz, W.K.: Nonmonotonic dose-response relationships: mechanistic basis, kinetic modeling, and implications for risk assessment. Toxicol. Sci. **77**(2), 151–157 (2004)

Cox, D.R.: Regression models and life-tables (with discussion). J. R. Stat. Soc. Series B **34**(2), 187–220 (1972)

Dale, J.R.: Global cross-ratio models for bivariate, discrete, ordered responses. Biometrics **42**(4), 909–917 (1986)

Dragalin, V., Fedorov, V.: Adaptive designs for dose-finding based on efficacy-toxicity response. J. Stat. Plan. Inference **136**(6), 1800–1823 (2006)

Dragalin, V., Fedorov, V., Wu, Y.: Two-stage design for dose-finding that accounts for both efficacy and safety. Stat. Med. **27**(25), 5156–5176 (2008)

Ezzalfani, M., Burzykowski, T., Paoletti, X.: Joint modelling of a binary and a continuous outcome measured at two cycles to determine the optimal dose. J. R. Stat. Soc. Ser. C Appl. Stat. **68**(2), 369–384 (2019)

Fan, S.K., Wang, Y.-G.: Decision-theoretic designs for dose-finding clinical trials with multiple outcomes. Stat. Med. **25**(10), 1699–1714 (2006)

Fedorov, V., Wu, Y.: Dose finding designs for continuous responses and binary utility. J. Biopharm. Stat. **17**(6), 1085–1096 (2007)

Guo, B., Li, Y., Yuan, Y.: A dose-schedule finding design for phase I–II clinical trials. J. R. Stat. Soc. Ser. C Appl. Stat. **65**(2), 259–272 (2016)

Guo, B., Yuan, Y.: Bayesian phase I/II biomarker-based dose finding for precision medicine with molecularly targeted agents. J. Amer. Stat. Assoc. **112**(518), 508–520 (2017)

Gooley, T.A., Martin, P.J., Fisher, L.D., Pettinger, M.: Simulation as a design tool for phase I/II clinical trials: an example from bone marrow transplantation. Control. Clin. Trials **15**(6), 450–462 (1994)

Hardwick, J., Meyer, M.C., Stout, Q.F.: Directed walk designs for dose response problems with competing failure modes. Biometrics **59**(2), 229–236 (2003)

Hirakawa, A.: An adaptive dose-finding approach for correlated bivariate binary and continuous outcomes in phase I oncology trials. Stat. Med. **31**(6), 516–532 (2012)

Hirakawa, A., Sato, H., Daimon, T., Matsui, S.: Modern Dose-Finding Designs for Cancer Phase I Trials: Drug Combinations and Molecularly Targeted Agents. Springer, Tokyo (2018)

Hoering, A., Mitchell, A., LeBlanc, M., Crowley, J.: Early phase trial design for assessing several dose levels for toxicity and efficacy for targeted agents. Clin. Trials **10**(3), 422–429 (2013)

Houede, N., Thall, P.F., Nguyen, H., Paoletti, X., Kramar, A.: Utility-based optimization of combination therapy using ordinal toxicity and efficacy in phase I/II trials. Biometrics **66**(2), 532–540 (2010)

Huang, X., Biswas, S., Oki, Y., Issa, J.-P., Berry, D.A.: A parallel phase I/II clinical trial design for combination therapies. Biometrics **63**(2), 429–436 (2007)

Hunsberger, S., Rubinstein, L.V., Dancey, J., Korn, E.L.: Dose escalation trial designs based on a molecularly targeted endpoint. Stat. Med. **24**(14), 2171–2181 (2005)

Ivanova, A.: A new dose-finding design for bivariate outcomes. Biometrics **59**(4), 1001–1007 (2003)

Ivanova, A., Liu, K., Snyder, E., Snavely, D.: An adaptive design for identifying the dose with the best efficacy/tolerability profile with application to a crossover dose-finding study. Stat. Med. **28**(24), 2941–2951 (2009)

Ji, Y., Liu, P., Li, Y., Bekele, B.N.: A modified toxicity probability interval method for dose-finding trials. Clin. Trials **7**(6), 653–663 (2010)

Kakurai, Y., Kaneko, S., Hamada, C., Hirakawa, A.: Dose individualization and variable selection by using the Bayesian lasso in early phase dose finding trials. J. R. Stat. Soc. Ser. C Appl. Stat. **68**(2), 445–460 (2019)

Kpamegan, E.E., Flournoy, N.: Chapter 19. An optimizing up-and-down design. In: Atkinson, A., Bogacka, B., Zhigljavsky, A. (eds.) Optimum Design 2000. Nonconvex Optimization and Its Applications, 1st edn, vol 51, pp. 211–224. Springer, Boston, MA (2001)

Lagarde, F., Beausoleil, C., Belcher, S.M., Belzunces, L.P., Emond, C., Guerbet, M., Rousselle, C.: Non-monotonic dose-response relationships and endocrine disruptors: a qualitative method of assessment. Environ. Health **14**(13), 1–13 (2015)

Le Tourneau, C., Dieras, V., Tresca, P., Cacheux, W., Paoletti, X.: Current challenges for the early clinical development of anticancer drugs in the era of molecularly targeted agents. Target Oncol. **5**(1), 65–72 (2010)

Leung, D., Wang, Y.-G.: An extension of the continual reassessment method using decision theory. Stat. Med. **21**(1), 51–63 (2002)

Li, Y., Bekele, B.N., Ji, Y., Cook, J.D.: Dose-schedule finding in phase I/II clinical trials using a Bayesian isotonic transformation. Stat. Med. **27**(24), 4895–4913 (2008)

Li, D.H., Whitmore, J.B., Guo, W., Ji, Y.: Toxicity and efficacy probability interval design for phase I adoptive cell therapy dose-finding clinical trials. Clin. Cancer Res. **23**(1), 13–20 (2016)

Liu, S., Johnson, V.E.: A robust Bayesian dose-finding design for phase I/II clinical trials. Biostatistics **17**(2), 249–263 (2016)

Liu, S., Yuan, Y.: Bayesian optimal interval designs for phase I clinical trials. J. Roy. Stat. Soc. Ser. C Appl. Stat. **64**(3), 507–523 (2015)

Loke, Y.-C., Tan, S.-B., Cai, Y.Y., Machin, D.: A Bayesian dose finding design for dual endpoint phase I trials. Stat. Med. **25**(1), 3–22 (2006)

Mandrekar, S.J., Cui, Y., Sargent, D.J.: An adaptive phase I design for identifying a biologically optimal dose for dual agent drug combinations. Stat. Med. **26**(11), 2317–2330 (2007)

Mandrekar, S.J., Qin, R., Sargent, D.J.: Model-based phase I designs incorporating toxicity and efficacy for single and dual agent drug combinations: methods and challenges. Stat. Med. **29**(10), 1077–1083 (2010)

Morgan, B., Thomas, A.L., Drevs, J., Hennig, J., Buchert, M., Jivan, A., Horsfield, M.A., Mross, K., Ball, H.A., Lee, L., Mietlowski, W., Fuxuis, S., Unger, C., O'Byrne, K., Henry, A., Cherryman, G., Laurent, D., Dugan, M., Marmé, D., Steward, W.: Dynamic contrast enhanced magnetic resonance imaging as a biomarker for the pharmacological response of ptk787/zk 222584, an inhibitor of the vascular endothelial growth factor receptor tyrosine kinases, in patients with advanced colorectal cancer and liver metastases: results from two phase I studies. J. Clin. Oncol. **21**(21), 3955–3964 (2003)

Mozgunov, P., Jaki, T.: An information theoretic phase I–II design for molecularly targeted agents that does not require an assumption of monotonicity. J. Roy. Stat. Soc. Ser. C Appl. Stat. **68**(2), 347–367 (2019)

Muenz, D.G., Taylor, J.M.G., Braun, T.M.: Phase I–II trial design for biologic agents using conditional auto-regressive models for toxicity and efficacy. J. R. Stat. Soc. Ser. C Appl. Stat. **68**(2), 331–345 (2019)

Murtaugh, P.A., Fisher, L.D.: Bivariate binary models of efficacy and toxicity in dose-ranging trials. Commun. Stat. Theory Methods **19**(6), 2003–2020 (1990)

O'Quigley, J., Hughes, M.D., Fenton, T.: Dose-finding designs for HIV studies. Biometrics **57**(4), 1018–1029 (2001)

O'Quigley, J., Hughes, M.D., Fenton, T., Pei, L.: Dynamic calibration of pharmacokinetic parameters in dose-finding studies. Biostatistics 11(3), 537–545 (2010)

O'Quigley, J., Paoletti, X., Maccario, J.: Non-parametric optimal design in dose finding studies. Biostatistics 3(1), 51–56 (2002)

O'Quigley, J., Shen, L.Z.: Continual reassessment method: a likelihood approach. Biometrics 52(2), 673–684 (1996)

Patterson, S., Francis, S., Ireson, M., Webber, D., Whitehead, J.: A novel Bayesian decision procedure for early-phase dose-finding studies. J. Biopharm. Stat. 9(4), 583–597 (1999)

Padmanabhan, S.K., Hsuan, F., Dragalin, V.: Adaptive penalized D-optimal designs for dose finding based on continuous efficacy and toxicity. Stat. Biopharm. Res. 2(2), 182–198 (2010)

Paoletti, X., Le Tourneau, C., Verweij, J., Siu, L.L., Seymour, L., Postel-Vinay, S., Collette, L., Rizzo, E., Ivy, P., Olmos, D., Massard, C., Lacombe, D., Kaye, S.B., Soria, J.C.: Defining dose-limiting toxicity for phase 1 trials of molecularly targeted agents: results of a DLT-TARGETT international survey. Eur. J. Cancer 50(12), 2050–2056 (2014)

Polley, M.-Y., Cheung, Y.K.: Two-stage designs for dose-finding trials with a biologic endpoint using stepwise tests. Biometrics 64(1), 232–241 (2008)

Postel-Vinay, S., Gomez-Roca, C., Molife, L.R., Anghan, B., Levy, A., Judson, I., De Bono, J., Soria, J.-C., Kaye, S., Paoletti, X.: Phase I trials of molecularly targeted agents: should we pay more attention to late toxicities? J. Clin. Oncol. 29(13), 1728–1735 (2011)

Pronzato, L.: Penalized optimal designs for dose-finding. J. Stat. Plan. Inference 140(1), 283–296 (2010)

Riviere, M.K., Yuan, Y., Dubois, F., Zohar, S.: A Bayesian dose finding design for clinical trials combining a cytotoxic agent with a molecularly targeted agent. J. Roy. Stat. Soc. Ser. C Appl. Stat. 64(1), 215–229 (2015)

Riviere, M.K., Yuan, Y., Jourdan, J.H., Dubois, F., Zohar, S.: Phase I/II dose-finding design for molecularly targeted agent: plateau determination using adaptive randomization. Stat. Methods Med. Res. 27(2), 466–479 (2018)

Robert, C., Ribas, A., Wolchok, J.D., Hodi, F.S., Hamid, O., Kefford, R., Weber, J.S., Joshua, A.M., Hwu, W.-J., Gangadhar, T.C.: Anti-programmed-death-receptor-1 treatment with pembrolizumab in ipilimumab refractory advanced melanoma: a randomised dose comparison cohort of a phase 1 trial. Lancet 384(9948), 1109–1117 (2014)

Storer, B.E.: Design and analysis of phase I clinical trials. Biometrics 45(3), 925–937 (1989)

Takeda, K., Taguri, M., Morita, S.: BOIN-ET: Bayesian optimal interval design for dose finding based on both efficacy and toxicity outcomes. Pharm. Stat. 17(4), 383–395 (2018)

Thall, P.F., Cheng, S.C.: Treatment comparisons based on two-dimensional safety and efficacy alternatives in oncology trials. Biometrics 55(3), 746–753 (1999)

Thall, P.F., Cook, J.D.: Dose-finding based on efficacy-toxicity trade-offs. Biometrics 60(3), 684–693 (2004)

Thall, P.F., Inoue, L.Y.T., Martin, T.G.: Adaptive decision making in a lymphocyte infusion trial. Biometrics 58(3), 560–568 (2002)

Thall, P.F., Nguyen, H.Q., Estey, E.H.: Patient-specific dose finding based on bivariate outcomes and covariates. Biometrics 64(4), 1126–1136 (2008)

Thall, P.F., Russell, K.E.: A strategy for dose-finding and safety monitoring based on efficacy and adverse outcomes in phase I/II clinical trials. Biometrics 54(1), 251–264 (1998)

Thall, P.F., Sung, H.-G., Choudhury, A.: Dose-finding based on feasibility and toxicity in T-cell infusion trials. Biometrics 57(3), 914–921 (2001)

Wages, N.A., Tait, C.: Seamless phase I/II adaptive design for oncology trials of molecularly targeted agents. J. Biopharm. Stat. 25(5), 903–920 (2015)

Wang, M., Day, R.: Adaptive Bayesian design for phase I dose-finding trials using a joint model of response and toxicity. J. Biopharm. Stat. 20(1), 125–144 (2010)

Whitehead, J., Brunier, H.: Bayesian decision procedures for dose determining experiments. Stat. Med. 14(9), 885–893 (1995)

Whitehead, J., Thygesen, H., Whitehead, A.: A Bayesian dose-finding procedure for phase I clinical trials based only on the assumption of monotonicity. Stat. Med. **29**(17), 1808–1824 (2010)

Whitehead, J., Thygesen, H., Whitehead, A.: Bayesian procedures for phase I/II clinical trials investigating the safety and efficacy of drug combinations. Stat. Med. **30**(16), 1952–1970 (2011)

Whitehead, J., Zhou, Y., Patterson, S., Webber, D., Francis, S.: Easy-to-implement Bayesian methods for dose-escalation studies in healthy volunteers. Biostatistics **2**(1), 47–61 (2001)

Whitehead, J., Zhou, Y., Stevens, J., Blakey, G.: An evaluation of a Bayesian method of dose-escalation based on bivariate binary responses. J. Biopharm. Stat. **14**(4), 969–983 (2004)

Whitehead, J., Zhou, Y., Mander, A., Ritchie, S., Sabin, A., Wright, A.: An evaluation of Bayesian designs for dose-escalation studies in healthy volunteers. Stat. Med. **25**(3), 433–445 (2006a)

Whitehead, J., Zhou, Y., Stevens, J., Blakey, G., Price, J., Leadbetter, J.: Bayesian decision procedures for dose-escalation based on evidence of undesirable events and therapeutic benefit. Stat. Med. **25**(1), 37–53 (2006b)

Yeung, W.Y., Reigner, B., Beyer, U., Diack, C., Sabanés Bové, D., Palermo, G. Jaki, T.: Bayesian adaptive dose-escalation designs for simultaneously estimating the optimal and maximum safe dose based on safety and efficacy. Pharm. Stat. **16**(6), 396–413 (2017)

Yeung, W.Y., Whitehead, J., Reigner, B., Beyer, U., Diack, C., Jaki, T.: Bayesian adaptive dose-escalation procedures for binary and continuous responses utilizing a gain function. Pharm. Stat. **14**(6), 479–487 (2015)

Yin, G., Li, Y., Ji, Y.: Bayesian dose-finding in phase I/II clinical trials using toxicity and efficacy odds ratios. Biometrics **62**(3), 777–787 (2006)

Yin, G., Zheng, S., Xu, J.: Two-stage dose finding for cytostatic agents in phase I oncology trials. Stat. Med. **32**(4), 644–660 (2013)

Yuan, Y., Yin, G.: Bayesian dose finding by jointly modelling toxicity and efficacy as time-to-event outcomes. J. R. Stat. Soc. Ser. C Appl. Stat. **58**(5), 719–736 (2009)

Zang, Y., Lee, J.J., Yuan, Y.: Adaptive designs for identifying optimal biological dose for molecularly targeted agents. Clin. Trials **11**(3), 319–327 (2014)

Zelen, M.: Play the winner rule and the controlled clinical trial. J. Amer. Stat. Assoc. **64**(325), 131–146 (1969)

Zhang, W., Sargent, D.J., Mandrekar, S.: An adaptive dose-finding design incorporating both toxicity and efficacy. Stat. Med. **25**(14), 2365–2383 (2006)

Zhou, Y., Whitehead, J., Bonvini, E., Stevens, J.: Bayesian decision procedures for binary and continuous bivariate dose-escalation studies. Pharm. Stat. **5**(2), 125–133 (2006)

Zohar, S., O'Quigley, J.: Identifying the most successful dose (MSD) in dose-finding studies in cancer. Pharm. Stat. **5**(3), 187–199 (2006a)

Zohar, S., O'Quigley, J.: Optimal designs for estimating the most successful dose. Stat. Med. **25**(24), 4311–4320 (2006b)

Chapter 6
Designs for Early-Phase Immunotherapeutic Agent Trials

Abstract Cancer immunotherapy is a broad category of anticancer therapies that induce, enhance, or suppress the immune system of a patient to help beat cancer. This therapy can also be regarded as a type of biological therapy that uses substances made from living organisms to treat cancer, because it employs white blood cells and organs and tissues of the lymph system. Therefore, in cancer immunotherapy, determination of biologically optimal doses is critical to successful treatment. Such doses are found by considering the outcome related to the immune response in addition to the toxicity and efficacy outcomes. This chapter reviews several dose-finding designs for early-phase immunotherapy trials.

Keywords Cancer immunotherapy · Immune response · Risk-benefit trade-off design · Seamless phase I/II randomized design · Dose expansion cohorts

6.1 Introduction

Recently, immunotherapy has attracted considerable attention as a cancer treatment option (Couzin-Frankel 2013). Immunotherapy helps the human immune system directly attack cancer and involves, e.g., checkpoint inhibitors, adaptive cell transfer, monoclonal antibodies, vaccines, and cytokines. Because the immune system recognizes and attacks the target tumor, immunotherapy is more personalized than molecularly targeted therapies. The key to successful immunotherapy is to determine the optimal dose (OD) of the agent administered to the patient. However, as for molecularly targeted agents (MTAs), conventional phase I trials considering toxicity alone (see Chaps. 2–4) for chemotherapeutic agents (CAs) may not be suitable in the case of immunotherapeutic agents (IAs), although unfortunately, they have often been used in practice, sometimes including dose expansion cohorts (see Sect. 6.5). In fact, as shown by Morrissey et al. (2016), MTD identification has not been successfully achieved for single-agent phase I trials involving nivolmub, pembrolizumab, and iplimumab. In addition, note that, in phase I trials of cancer vaccines, this failure commonly occurs because of the flat dose–toxicity relationship. Furthermore, the assumption that the efficacy monotonically increases with increasing dose

© The Author(s), under exclusive licence to Springer Japan KK 2019
T. Daimon et al., *Dose-Finding Designs for Early-Phase Cancer Clinical Trials*, JSS Research Series in Statistics, https://doi.org/10.1007/978-4-431-55585-8_6

may be inappropriate for IAs, because the mechanism of action for immunotherapies is based on enhancement of the immune system. Therefore, phase I/II trial designs considering toxicity, efficacy, and immune response are recommended for IA dose optimization. We overview some of these designs. In particular, for cancer therapeutic vaccine trials, see, e.g., Cunanan and Koopmeiners (2017) and Wang et al. (2018).

6.2 Toxicity Evaluation Design

Messer et al. (2010) proposed a toxicity evaluation (estimation) design for phase I/II cancer immunotherapy trials. This design is based on safety hypothesis testing and an algorithm similar to a $3 + 3$ design. For the first basis, given a target toxicity probability level, the design allows testing of a one-sided null hypothesis. That is, for the null hypothesis, the toxicity rate is taken to be inadmissibly high if the data do not provide evidence to the contrary. For the alternative hypothesis, it may be established that the toxicity rate is admissible if the observed toxicity rate is too low to support the null hypothesis. For the second basis, in the phase I trial part, all patient cohorts are treated with one proposed therapeutic dose (that is, there is no dose escalation). Further, each cohort is either small (three patients) or expanded (six patients), similar to a $3 + 3$ design. Specifically, the $3 + 3$ design algorithm is adapted as follows: if at least two of the three patients experience toxicity, the trial is terminated. If none of the three patients experience toxicity, the next cohort is enrolled and treated. If one of the three patients experiences toxicity, the current cohort is expanded by three more patients. If none of these three patients experience toxicity (that is, only one patient of the six total experiences toxicity), the trial is continued, and the next cohort is enrolled and treated. Alternatively, if at least one of these three patients experiences toxicity (i.e., two or more of the six total), the trial is terminated. Finally, if all cohorts archive the safety endpoint without trial closure, the phase I part is followed by the phase II part for efficacy assessment.

The therapeutic dose may be found after an initial dose escalation stage; thus, it may be desirable to use the toxicity estimation design as a second stage. Messer et al. (2010) gave the upper limit of an exact confidence interval for the toxicity rate at the therapeutic dose using the combined phase I and II trials' toxicity data, as well as the maximum likelihood estimate of the toxicity rate. Note that the toxicity estimation design works well only if the true toxicity rate is well below the acceptable toxicity rate.

6.3 Risk-Benefit Trade-off Design

Liu et al. (2018) proposed a phase I/II trial design to determine the biologically optimal dose (BOD) of an IA in which three outcomes are simultaneously considered: the immune response, toxicity, and efficacy. The BOD in this design is given by the dose yielding the highest desirability in the risk-benefit trade-off between the undesirable and desirable outcomes for the three outcomes, which is measured via a utility function to lay the multidimensional outcomes into a single index. Although we focus on the design of Liu et al. (2018), readers are also referred to Guo et al. (2019), who propose a novel design for immunotherapy trials called BDFIT to find the OBD. One difference between Liu et al. (2018) and Guo et al. (2019) is that the former considered the objective tumor response as the efficacy outcome, whereas the latter considered the progression-free survival as the efficacy outcome.

6.3.1 Probability Models

Suppose that, in a phase I/II trial with a prespecified maximum sample size n_{max}, we attempt to identify the BOD of an IA among its ordered doses $d_1 < \cdots < d_K$. Let Y_I denote the random variable for the immune response, such as the concentration of a cytokine or the T-cell count. Let Y_T denote the binary random variable for the toxicity outcome, where $Y_T = 1$ indicates toxicity, with $Y_T = 0$ otherwise. Let Y_E denote the trinary ordinal random variable for the efficacy outcome, where $Y_E = 0, 1$, and 2 indicate progressive disease (PD), stable disease (SD), and partial response (PR) or complete response (CR) as the objective tumor response, respectively. Traditionally, patients with CR or PR are regarded as responders, whereas those with SD or PD are not. However, in immuno-oncology, SD is often considered as a positive response, because patients with durable SD achieve long-term survival, even though they do not exhibit notable tumor shrinkage.

Liu et al. (2018) considered these three outcomes as a trinary vector, denoted by $Y = (Y_I, Y_T, Y_E)$. This approach is contrary to most existing phase I/II trial designs, which focus on (Y_T, Y_E) only. Liu et al. (2018) considered the fact that, in immunotherapy, toxicity and efficacy outcomes are activated by the immune system, and employed the following probability modeling.

The joint distribution of (Y_I, Y_T, Y_E) given dose d, denoted by $[Y_I, Y_T, Y_E|d]$, is factorized into the product of the marginal distribution of Y_I given dose d, denoted by $[Y_I|d]$, and the conditional distribution of (Y_T, Y_E) given d and Y_I, denoted by $[Y_T, Y_E|d, Y_I]$. That is,

$$[Y_I, Y_T, Y_E|d] = [Y_I|d][Y_T, Y_E|d, Y_I]. \tag{6.1}$$

The marginal distribution $[Y_I|d]$ is modeled using an E_{max} model, which is a non-linear model frequently used to elucidate a dose–response relationship, as follows:

$$Y_I = \beta_0 + \frac{\beta_1 d^{\beta_3}}{\beta_2^{\beta_3} + d^{\beta_3}} + \varepsilon, \tag{6.2}$$

where β_0 is the baseline immune activity corresponding to the activity when the dose of the IA is zero; β_1 is the maximum immune activity attributable to the IA, often denoted as E_{max}; β_2 is the dose that yields half of the maximum immune activity, often denoted as ED_{50}; β_3 is the slope factor, also called the Hill factor, which measures the response sensitivity to the IA dose range, controlling the steepness of the dose–activity curve; and ε is the error that is assumed to have normal distribution with a mean of 0 and variance σ^2, denoted by $\varepsilon \sim N(0, \sigma^2)$. The joint distribution $[Y_T, Y_E | d, Y_I]$ is modeled using a latent variable model, which allows a set of directly observable variables (manifest variables) to be related to a set of directly unobservable variables (latent variables). Let Z_T and Z_E denote two continuous latent variables related to manifest variables Y_T and Y_E, respectively, as follows:

$$Y_T = \begin{cases} 0 \text{ if } Z_T < \zeta_1 \\ 1 \text{ if } Z_T \geq \zeta_1 \end{cases} \text{ and } Y_E = \begin{cases} 0 \text{ if } Z_E < \eta_1 \\ 1 \text{ if } \eta_1 \leq Z_T < \eta_2 \ , \\ 2 \text{ if } Z_E \geq \eta_2 \end{cases} \tag{6.3}$$

where ζ_1, η_1, and η_2 are unknown cutpoints. It is assumed that $[Z_T, Z_E | Y_I, d]$ is bivariate normally distributed with mean vector μ and variance–covariance matrix Σ, denoted by $(Z_T, Z_E)^T \sim BN(\mu, \Sigma)$, where

$$\mu = \begin{pmatrix} \mu_T(Y_I, d) \\ \mu_E(Y_I, d) \end{pmatrix} \text{ and } \Sigma = \begin{pmatrix} \sigma_{11} & \sigma_{12} \\ \sigma_{12} & \sigma_{22} \end{pmatrix}. \tag{6.4}$$

Further, $\mu_l(Y_I, d) = E(Z_l | Y_I, d)$ is the expectation of Z_l, conditional on Y_I and d, for $l = T$ or E; and σ_{11}, σ_{12}, and σ_{22} are unknown parameters. However, to identify the model, $\zeta_1 = \eta_1 = 0$ and $\sigma_{11} = \sigma_{22} = 1$, with the constraint $0 \leq \sigma_{12} \leq 1$.

The model for $\mu_T(Y_I, d)$ is given by

$$\mu_T(Y_I, d) = \beta_4 + \beta_5 d + I(Y_I > \beta_7)\beta_6 Y_I, \tag{6.5}$$

where β_4, β_5, β_6, and β_7 are unknown parameters. In addition, $I(Y_I > \beta_7)$ is the indicator function, having a value of 1 if $Y_I > \beta_7$ and 0 otherwise. Under this model, d is included as a covariate to capture the possible relationship between the dose and toxicity, and Y_I does not induce toxicity unless it exceeds the β_7 threshold.

The model for $\mu_E(Y_I, d)$ is given by

$$\mu_E(Y_I, d) = \beta_8 + \beta_9 Y_I + \beta_{10} Y_I^2, \tag{6.6}$$

where β_8, β_9, and β_{10} are unknown parameters. Under this model, Y_E is independent of d, conditional on Y_I, because the efficacy can be produced by mediation of the immune response. In addition, the quadratic term Y_I^2 is used to take into account the possibility that the efficacy may not monotonically increase with Y_I. It should be noted that this model is regarded as a working model to obtain a reasonable local fit for guidance of the dose-finding process, rather than accurate estimation of the entire immune-response curve. Liu et al. (2018) showed that this model works reasonably well even in the scenario where the true immune-response curve has an increasing trend followed by a plateau shape, which is often encountered in practice.

For the ith patient, let $\mathbf{y}_i = (y_{I,i}, y_{T,i}, y_{E,i})$ denote the observed value for $\mathbf{Y}_i = (Y_{I,i}, Y_{T,i}, Y_{E,i})$; $d_{[i]}$ the assigned dose, for $i = 1, \ldots, n_{\max}$; and $\boldsymbol{\beta}$ the vector of parameters, denoted by $\boldsymbol{\beta} = (\boldsymbol{\beta}_1 | \boldsymbol{\beta}_2) = (\beta_0, \ldots, \beta_3 | \beta_4, \ldots, \beta_7)$, where $\boldsymbol{\beta}_1$ and $\boldsymbol{\beta}_2$ are subvectors of $\boldsymbol{\beta}$. Defining $\zeta_0 = \eta_0 \equiv -\infty$ and $\zeta_2 = \eta_3 \equiv \infty$, the likelihood for the manifest variables for the ith patient is given by

$$
\begin{aligned}
\mathcal{L}(\mathbf{y}_i | d_{[i]}, \boldsymbol{\beta}) &= f(y_{I,i} | d_{[i]}, \boldsymbol{\beta}_1) \Pr(Y_{T,i} = y_{T,i}, Y_{E,i} = y_{E,i} | y_{I,i}, d_{[i]}, \boldsymbol{\beta}_2) \\
&= f(y_{I,i} | d_{[i]}, \boldsymbol{\beta}_1) \\
&\quad \times \Pr(\zeta_{y_{T,i}} \le Z_{T,i} < \zeta_{y_{T,i+1}}, \eta_{y_{E,i}} \le Z_{E,i} < \eta_{y_{E,i+1}} | y_{I,i}, d_{[i]}, \boldsymbol{\beta}_2) \\
&= f(y_{I,i} | d_{[i]}, \boldsymbol{\beta}_1) \\
&\quad \times \int_{\zeta_{y_{T,i}}}^{\zeta_{y_{T,i+1}}} \int_{\eta_{y_{E,i}}}^{\eta_{y_{E,i+1}}} f(Z_{T,i}, Z_{E,i} | y_{I,i}, d_{[i]}, \boldsymbol{\beta}_2) \mathrm{d}Z_{T,i} \mathrm{d}Z_{E,i}, \quad (6.7)
\end{aligned}
$$

where $f(y_{I,i} | d_{[i]}, \boldsymbol{\beta}_1)$ is the probability density function of $Y_{I,i}$ given $d_{[i]}$, with the subvector parameter $\boldsymbol{\beta}_1$; and $f(Z_{T,i}, Z_{E,i} | Y_{I,i}, d_{[i]}, \boldsymbol{\beta}_2)$ is the probability density function of $(Z_{T,i}, Z_{E,i})$, conditional on $Y_{I,i}$ and $d_{[i]}$, with the subvector parameter $\boldsymbol{\beta}_2$. Let $n = 1, \ldots, n_{\max}$ represent the interim sample size when a decision on dose escalation, de-escalation, or maintenance for the next patient or cohort of patients is to be made during the trial. Further, $\mathfrak{D}_n = (\mathbf{y}, \ldots, \mathbf{y}_n)$ represent the data observed from the first n patients. Then, the likelihood for the first n patients in the trial is $\mathcal{L}(\mathfrak{D}_n | \boldsymbol{\beta}) = \prod_{i=1}^{n} \mathcal{L}(\mathbf{y} | d_{[i]}, \boldsymbol{\beta})$. Let $p(\boldsymbol{\beta})$ denote the joint prior distribution of $\boldsymbol{\beta}$. The joint posterior distribution based on the data from the first n patients is $p(\boldsymbol{\beta} | \mathfrak{D}_n) \propto \mathcal{L}_n(\mathfrak{D}_n | \boldsymbol{\beta}) p(\boldsymbol{\beta})$. See Liu et al. (2018) for the prior specification of $\boldsymbol{\beta}$.

6.3.2 Dose-Finding Algorithm

6.3.2.1 Definition of Optimal Dose

Liu et al. (2018) proposed use of a utility function to identify the BOD based on trade-offs among the immune response, efficacy, and toxicity considered desirable by clinicians or patients. The utility function allows mapping of the multidimensional outcomes into a single index for the dose desirability, and has been used in most dose-finding designs (see, e.g., Houede et al. 2010; Thall et al. 2013, 2014; Yuan et al. 2016; Guo and Yuan 2017).

Let $U(Y_I, Y_T, Y_E)$ denote a utility function. Liu et al. (2018) presented a convenient method of eliciting $U(Y_I, Y_T, Y_E)$ as follows: (1) the immune response Y_I is dichotomized as desirable ($\tilde{Y}_I = 1$) or undesirable ($\tilde{Y}_I = 0$) based on a certain cutoff value specified by the clinicians, or can be categorized into more than three levels; (2) The scores of the least (i.e., the undesirable immune response, toxicity, and PD) and most (i.e., the desirable immune response, an absence of toxicity, and CR/PR) desirable outcomes are fixed as $U(\tilde{Y}_1, Y_T, Y_E) = 0$ and $U(\tilde{Y}_1, Y_T, Y_E) = 100$, respectively. Then, using these two scores as boundaries, the scores of other possible outcomes are elicited from the clinical investigators, such that they are located between 0 and 100.

For a given dose d, the corresponding utility $U(d)$ is given by

$$E(U(d)|\boldsymbol{\beta}) = \int U(\tilde{Y}_1, Y_T, Y_E) f(\tilde{Y}_1, Y_T, Y_E) d\tilde{Y}_1 dY_T dY_E, \qquad (6.8)$$

where $f(\tilde{Y}_1, Y_T, Y_E)$ is a probability function for $(\tilde{Y}_1, Y_T, Y_E)$. However, because $\boldsymbol{\beta}$ is unknown, the utility of d must be estimated. Specifically, given interim data $\mathfrak{D}_n$, the utility of d is estimated from its posterior mean

$$E(U(d)|\mathfrak{D}_n) = \int E(U(d)|\boldsymbol{\beta}) p(\boldsymbol{\beta}|\mathfrak{D}_n) d\boldsymbol{\beta}. \qquad (6.9)$$

This posterior mean utility is used to evaluate the desirability of a certain dose and to guide dose finding. However, a dose that is optimal in terms of utility alone may not be acceptable with regard to either toxicity or efficacy. Therefore, the OD in this design is defined as that having the highest utility while satisfying the acceptable toxicity and efficacy requirements (for details, see Liu et al. 2018).

6.3.2.2 Dose-Finding Algorithm

Suppose that patients are treated in cohorts of size m with an interim sample size of $n = m \times r$. Consequently, the maximum sample size is $n_{max} = m \times R$, where r is the number of cohorts, for $r = 1, \ldots, R - 1$. Let d_h denote the current highest tested dose, and $\mathfrak{A}_n$ the set of admissible doses, which are defined as those satisfying the acceptable toxicity and efficacy requirements, for a given interim sample size n. The first patient cohort is treated at the lowest dose d_1. The following dose-finding algorithm is used for treatment of the $(r+1)$th cohort of patients at a given dose (for details, see Liu et al. 2018):

Step 1   If $\mathfrak{D}_n$ shows that d_h is safe, we continue dose-finding by treating the $(r+1)$th cohort at the next highest new dose d_{h+1}.

Step 2   Otherwise, we identify $\mathfrak{A}_n$ and adaptively randomize the $(r+1)$th cohort to dose $d_k \in \mathfrak{A}_n$ (k=1,...,K), with probability

$$\Pr(U(d_k) = \max\{U(d_{k'}), k' \in \mathfrak{A}_n\} | \mathfrak{D}_n), \qquad (6.10)$$

and Eq. (6.10) represents the posterior probability that dose level k is the level with the highest posterior mean utility. If $\mathfrak{A}_n$ is empty, the trial is terminated.

Step 3   Once n_{max} is achieved, the dose in $\mathfrak{A}_{n_{max}}$ with the highest posterior mean utility is recommended.

6.3.3 Summary of Operating Characteristics

Liu et al. (2018) illustrated the behavior of their dose-finding design in a simulation study involving eight scenarios that varied with regard to the true dose-response relationships for toxicity, efficacy, and immune response. They considered five doses with a maximum sample size of 60 in a cohort size of 3, and compared their design with a phase I/II trial design that considers efficacy and toxicity only, namely, the "EffTox design" proposed by Thall and Cook (2004). The utility used in the EffTox design was obtained by averaging $U(Y_I, Y_T, Y_E)$ over Y_I. As a result, in seven scenarios including ODs, the design proposed by Liu et al. (2018) outperformed the EffTox design with respect to the percentage of correctly selected ODs and the number of patients to which the OD was assigned. In addition, those researchers also performed sensitivity analyses to evaluate the robustness of their proposed design using a smaller sample size of 42, another set of utility values, different values for the prior estimates of the parameters in Eq. (6.2), and different prior distributions. Hence, they showed that their proposed design is not sensitive to any of these factors.

6.4 SPIRIT

Guo et al. (2018) proposed a seamless phase I/II randomized design for immunotherapy trials (SPIRIT) to determine the BOD of an IA. One important difference is that this design considers progression-free survival (PFS) as the efficacy outcome; in contrast, the above risk-benefit trade-off design, proposed by Liu et al. (2018), considers the ordinal objective tumor response as the efficacy outcome. The PFS takes a relatively long time to observe and, thus, makes immediate adaptive dose assignment decisions hard, although the tumor response takes a relatively short time to observe, and thus makes immediate adaptive dose assignment decisions easy. As a consequence, the SPIRIT uses the immune response as an ancillary outcome to screen out inefficacious doses and to guess the PFS when necessary.

6.4.1 Probability Models

Suppose that, in a phase I/II trial with a prespecified maximum sample size $n_{\max}$, we attempt to identify the BOD of an IA among its ordered doses $d_1 < \cdots < d_K$. Let T_E denote the random variable for the PFS as the efficacy outcome, and t_E denote the observed value for T_E. Let Y_I denote the dichotomized random variable for the immune response, and y_I denote the observed value for Y_I. Here, $Y_I = 1$ if a patient has an immune response and 0 otherwise. Even if Y_I is continuous, extension of the following modeling approach is straightforward.

Guo et al. (2018) considered the following probability models. They assumed that, for dose level $k(= 1, \ldots, K)$, Y_I follows a Bernoulli distribution with parameter $\pi_{I,k} = \Pr(Y_I = 1|d_k)$. This parameter is the probability of a patient having an immune response at d_k. The random variable for the PFS (T_E) is modeled by Y_I using a proportional hazards model, conditional on the immune response Y_I and dose d_k. Specifically, let $h(t_E|y_I, d_k)$ indicate the PFS hazard function. That is, given immune response y_I and treated dose d_k, T_E is given by using the following proportional hazards model:

$$h(t_E|y_I, d_k) = h_0(t_E|d_k)\exp(\beta y_I), \tag{6.11}$$

where $h_0(t_E|d_k)$ is the baseline hazard at d_k and β is an unknown parameter. Here, it is assumed that T_E follows the Pareto distribution with shape parameter $\alpha > 0$ and scale parameter $\phi > 0$, because some patients receiving immunotherapy may produce long-term durable responses; thus, the PFS curve tends to be heavy tailed. Therefore, Eq. (6.11) is rewritten as

$$h(t_E|y_I, d_k) = \frac{\alpha_k}{t_E + \phi_k}\exp(\beta y_I), \tag{6.12}$$

where (α_k, ϕ_k) are the parameters of the Pareto distribution at d_k. That means that there is no structure in the relationship between the dose and PFS because the parameter is specified for each dose level.

Let n_k and $n_{I,k}$ denote the interim sample size and the number of patients having an immune response at dose level k, respectively, when a decision on dose escalation, de-escalation, or maintenance for the next patient or cohort of patients is to be made during the trial. For the ith treated patient, for $i = 1, \ldots, n_k$, let $t_{E,i}^o$ denote the observed event or censoring time. Further, let $\delta_i = I(T_{E,i}^o = T_{E,i})$ denote an indicator function regarding the event or censoring; this term takes a value of 1 when disease progression or death is observed at the time of $t_{E,i}^o$, that is, $t_{E,i}^o = t_{E,i}$, and 0 otherwise. The likelihood of the interim data $\mathfrak{D}_k = \{(t_{E,i}^o, \delta_i, y_{I,i})\}$ obtained at dose level k is given by

$$\mathfrak{L}(\mathfrak{D}_k|\alpha_k, \phi_k, \pi_{I,k}, \beta) = \prod_{i=1}^{n_k}\left\{f(y_{I,i}|\pi_{I,k})f(t_{E,i}^0|y_{I,i}, \alpha_k, \phi_k, \beta)^{\delta_i}S(t_{E,i}^0|y_{I,i}, \alpha_k, \phi_k, \beta)^{1-\delta_i}\right\}$$

$$= \pi_{I,k}^{n_{I,k}}(1 - \pi_{I,k})^{n_k - n_{I,k}}\prod_{i=1}^{n_k}\frac{\phi_k^{\alpha_k\exp(\beta y_{I,i})}\left\{\alpha_k\exp(\beta y_{I,i})\right\}^{\delta_i}}{(t_{E,i}^o + \phi_k)^{\alpha_k\exp(\beta y_{I,i})+\delta_i}}, \tag{6.13}$$

where $f(y_{I,i}|\pi_{I,k})$ is the probability density function of $Y_{I,i}$ with parameter $\pi_{I,k}$, and $f(t_{E,i}^0|y_{I,i}, \alpha_k, \phi_k, \beta)$ and $S(t_{E,i}^0|y_{I,i}, \alpha_k, \phi_k, \beta)$ are the probability density function and survival function of $T_{E,i}^0$ with parameters α_k, ϕ_k, and β, conditional on $Y_{I,i}$, respectively. The likelihood of the interim data $\mathfrak{D} = \{\mathfrak{D}_k\}$ that are obtained across all dose levels is given by

$$\mathfrak{D} = \prod_{k=1}^{K} \mathcal{L}(\mathfrak{D}_k | \alpha_k, \phi_k, \pi_{\mathrm{I},k}, \beta). \tag{6.14}$$

Guo et al. (2018) did not consider the joint distribution of the toxicity and efficacy, and modeled the marginal distribution of toxicity using a beta-binomial model to monitor safety. This is because, for immunotherapy, the efficacy may not be associated with toxicity, and in addition because consideration of this distribution does not necessarily improve the dose-finding performance (Cai et al. 2014).

Let $\pi_{\mathrm{T},k}$ denote the toxicity probability at dose level k. Suppose that, $n_{\mathrm{T},k}$ out of n_k patients experience toxicity. Then, the beta-binomial model is given by

$$n_{\mathrm{T},k} \sim \mathrm{Bin}(n_k, \pi_{\mathrm{T},k}) \text{ and } \pi_{\mathrm{T},k} \sim \mathrm{Beta}(a, b), \tag{6.15}$$

where a and b are hyperparameters. The posterior distribution of $\pi_{\mathrm{T},k}$ is also the beta distribution based on the conjugate analysis, denoted by $\mathrm{Beta}(a + n_{\mathrm{T},k}, b + n_k - n_{\mathrm{T},k})$.

Let $p(\boldsymbol{\beta})$ denote the prior distribution of $\boldsymbol{\beta} = \{\alpha_k, \phi_k, \beta, \pi_{\mathrm{I},k}; k = 1, \ldots, K\}$; $n = 1, \ldots, n_{\max}$ represent an interim sample size for which a decision on dose escalation, de-escalation, or maintenance for the next patient or cohort of patients is to be made during the trial; and $\mathfrak{D}_n$ indicate the data observed for the first n patients. The likelihood for the first n patients in the trial is $\mathcal{L}(\mathfrak{D}_n | \boldsymbol{\beta}) = \prod_{i=1}^{n} \mathcal{L}(\boldsymbol{y} | d_{[i]}, \boldsymbol{\beta})$, where $d_{[i]}$ is the dose administered for the treatment of ith patient. Then, the posterior distribution based on the data obtained from the first n patients is $p(\boldsymbol{\beta} | \mathfrak{D}_n) \propto \mathcal{L}(\mathfrak{D}_n | \boldsymbol{\beta}) p(\boldsymbol{\beta})$.

It is assumed that α_k and ϕ_k follow independent gamma prior distributions with hyperparameters $(\hat{\alpha}_k, \sigma_\alpha^2)$ and $(\hat{\phi}_k, \sigma_\phi^2)$, denoted by $\mathrm{Ga}(\hat{\alpha}_k, \sigma_\alpha^2)$ and $\mathrm{Ga}(\hat{\phi}_k, \sigma_\phi^2)$, respectively, where each gamma prior distribution is parameterized such that its first and second hyperparameters are the mean and variance, respectively. The mean hyperparameters $\hat{\alpha}_k$ and $\hat{\phi}_k$ are elicited from the clinical investigators. Specifically, they are asked to give estimates of the median PFS, denoted by M_k^*, and the proportion of patients with no disease progression at time τ, denoted by $S_k^*(\tau)$. Specifically, the following two equations are then solved to obtain $\hat{\alpha}_k$ and $\hat{\phi}_k$:

$$M_k^* = \phi_k(2^{1/\alpha_k} - 1), \tag{6.16}$$

$$S_k^*(\tau) = \left(\frac{\phi_k}{\tau + \phi_k}\right)^{\alpha_k}. \tag{6.17}$$

The variance hyperparameters σ_α^2 and σ_ϕ^2 are made relatively large so that the priors are vague. The prior of β is a uniform distribution, denoted by $\beta \sim \mathrm{U}((\log(r_1), \log(r_2)))$, where (r_1, r_2) is the range of the corresponding log hazard ratio of the PFS for the presence versus absence of immune response. The prior distribution of $\pi_{\mathrm{I},k}$ is a beta prior distribution with hyperparameters $\hat{\pi}_{\mathrm{I},k}$ and $\sigma_{\beta,k}^2$, where $\hat{\pi}_{\mathrm{I},k}$ is the prior estimate of the immune response elicited from the clinical investigators and $\sigma_{\beta,k}^2 = \hat{\pi}_{\mathrm{I},k}(1 - \hat{\pi}_{\mathrm{I},k})/2$. Thus, the beta prior is vague and has a prior effective sample size of one patient.

6.4.2 Dose-Finding Algorithm

6.4.2.1 Definition of Optimal Dose

Guo et al. (2018) proposed use of a restricted mean survival time (RMST) given as the area under the PFS curve, so as to measure the desirability of a certain dose or to compare desirability between doses. The RMST is an alternative to using the median PFS. This approach was adopted because for immunotherapy, the PFS often has a heavy-tailed distribution, but the median PFS cannot consider this aspect. For example, suppose that the PFS curves have the same median PFS across all doses, but different tails (Guo et al. 2018). To consider this dose, we prefer the RMST to the median PFS. Let $S(t_E)$ denote the PFS function, and τ the follow-up time of clinical interest. Then, the RMST is defined by

$$R(\tau) = \int_0^\tau S(t_E)dt_E. \tag{6.18}$$

Because the survival function here is a Pareto survival function, the RMST at dose level k is given by

$$
\begin{aligned}
R_k(\tau) &= \int_0^\tau S(t)dt \\
&= \frac{\pi_{1,k}\phi_k^{\alpha_k \exp(\beta)}}{1 - \alpha_k \exp(\beta)} \left\{ (\tau + \phi_k)^{1-\alpha_k \exp(\beta)} - \phi_k^{1-\alpha_k \exp(\beta)} \right\} \\
&\quad + \frac{(1 - \pi_{1,k})\phi_k^{\alpha_k}}{1 - \alpha_k} \left\{ (\tau + \phi_k)^{1-\alpha_k} - \phi_k^{1-\alpha_k} \right\}.
\end{aligned} \tag{6.19}
$$

Therefore, the OD in this design is defined as the dose having the highest RMST value while satisfying the acceptable toxicity and immuno-response requirements (for details, see Guo et al. 2018).

6.4.2.2 Dose-Finding Algorithm

Guo et al. (2018) presented the following dose-finding algorithm with two stages:
  Stage 1 consists of the following algorithm:

Step 1 Treat the first patient or cohort of patients at the first dose level, and evaluate whether each experiences toxicity.

Step 2 At the current dose level k, use the Bayesian optimal interval design (see Sect. 4.4) to identify the doses having admissible toxicity.

Step 3 Repeat Step 2 until the prespecified sample size at stage 1 is reached, and then move on to stage 2.

At stage 2, enrolled patients are adaptively randomized to the admissible doses that satisfy the prespecified requirements on the toxicity, immuno-response, and the highest RMST (for details, see Guo et al. 2018).

6.4.3 Summary of Operating Characteristics

Guo et al. (2018) investigated the operating characteristics of SPIRIT in a simulation study considering 10 scenarios that varied in terms of the true dose-response relationships for toxicity, efficacy, and immune response. They considered five doses with a maximum sample size of 60 and a stage 1 sample size of 21 (in a cohort size of 3 in both stages), and compared their design with a conventional design consisting of two stages (Iasonos and O'Quigley 2016). In the conventional design, in the first stage, the CRM was used to estimate the MTD with a sample size of 21; then, in the second stage, cohort was expanded at the MTD and at the dose one level lower than the MTD, with a sample size of $(60 - 21)/2$ at each dose. The OD was chosen as the dose yielding the highest PFS at the end of the follow-up time of 12.

It was assumed that both the toxicity and immune response could be quickly evaluated after treatment. The toxicity upper bound was 0.3 and the immune-response lower bound was 0.15. The patient accrual was assumed to follow a Poisson distribution with a rate of 3 per month. The prior means were set as $\hat{\alpha}_k = 1$ and $\hat{\phi}_k = 4$ at dose level $k (= 1, \ldots, 5)$, and the prior standard deviations of α_k and ϕ_k were set to $\sigma_\alpha = 3$ and $\sigma_\phi = 12$, respectively. The prior estimate was set to $\hat{\pi}_{1,k} = 0.3$, with $\pi_{1,k} \sim \text{Beta}(0.3, 0.105)$, corresponding to a prior sample size of 1. The prior distribution of β was set to $U(-2.3, 0)$, to reflect the prior information that the hazard ratio is expected to be within $(0.1,1)$. The hyperparameters a and b were set to $a = 0.3$ and $b = 0.7$, respectively, corresponding to a prior sample size of 1. For details on other configurations, see Guo et al. (2018).

As a result, in most of the nine scenarios that included ODs, SPIRIT exhibited desirable operating characteristics and outperformed the conventional design with respect to the percentage of correctly selected ODs and the number of patients to which the OD was assigned. In addition, sensitivity analyses were performed to evaluate the robustness of the SPIRIT performance, by assuming that the true distribution of the PFS has a log-logistic or Weibull distribution rather than the Pareto distribution. Hence, Guo et al. (2018) showed that their proposed design is insensitive to the PFS distribution.

6.5 Dose Expansion Cohorts

Early-phase clinical trials in oncology are classically composed of a phase I trial with a small heterogeneous patient population designed to determine the MTD, followed by a disease-specific phase II trial in which antitumor activity is evaluated.

However, in recent years, this approach has been changing because technological advances have enabled identification of a large number of promising agents that require testing in clinical trials. Consequently, the need to evaluate antitumor activity as efficiently as possible during the drug development process has increased. Specifically, a phase I trial can now be designed by adding dose expansion cohorts, to confirm that the MTD has been established; to obtain preliminary evidence of efficacy; and to identify specific patient subgroups that may derive particular benefits from the investigational drug (Iasonos and O'Quigley 2013, 2015). Designs for early-phase trials including details of the dose expansion cohorts have been proposed by, e.g., Iasonos and O'Quigley (2016, 2017). For further information on the use of dose expansion cohorts, see the draft guidance provided by the Food and Drug Administration available from https://www.fdanews.com/ext/resources/files/2018/08-10-18-DraftGuidance.pdf?1533913620.

References

Cai, C., Yuan, Y., Ji, Y.: A Bayesian dose finding design for oncology clinical trials of combinational biological agents. J. Roy. Stat. Soc. Ser. C Appl. Stat. **63**(1), 159–173 (2014)

Couzin-Frankel, J.: Cancer immunotherapy. Science **324**(6165), 1432–1433 (2013)

Cunanan, K.M., Koopmeiners, J.S.: A Bayesian adaptive phase I-II trial design for optimizing the schedule of therapeutic cancer vaccines. Stat. Med. **36**(1), 43–53 (2017)

Guo, B., Yuan, Y.: Bayesian phase I/II biomarker-based dose finding for precision medicine with molecularly targeted agents. J. Am. Stat. Assoc. **112**(518), 508–520 (2017)

Guo, B., Li, D., Yuan, Y.: SPIRIT: A seamless phase I/II randomized design for immunotherapy trials. Pharm. Stat. **17**(5), 527–540 (2018)

Guo, B., Park, Y., Liu, S.: A utility-based Bayesian phase I-II design for immunotherapy trials with progression-free survival end point. J. R. Stat. Soc. Ser. C Appl. Stat. **68**(2), 411–425 (2019)

Houede, N., Thall, P.F., Nguyen, H., Paoletti, X., Kramar, A.: Utility-based optimization of combination therapy using ordinal toxicity and efficacy in phase I/II trials. Biometrics **66**(2), 532–540 (2010)

Iasonos, A., O'Quigley, J.: Design considerations for dose-expansion cohorts in phase I trials. J. Clin. Oncol. **31**(31), 4014–4021 (2013)

Iasonos, A., O'Quigley, J.: Early phase clinical trials-are dose expansion cohorts needed? Nat. Rev. Clin. Oncol. **12**(11), 626–628 (2015)

Iasonos, A., O'Quigley, J.: Dose expansion cohorts in phase I trials. Stat. Biopharm. Res. **8**(2), 161–170 (2016)

Iasonos, A., O'Quigley, J.: Sequential monitoring of phase I dose expansion cohorts. Stat. Med. **36**(2), 204–214 (2017)

Liu, S., Guo, B., Yuan, Y.: A Bayesian phase I/II trial design for immunotherapy. J. Am. Stat. Assoc. (2018). https://doi.org/10.1080/01621459.2017.1383260

Messer, K., Natarajan, L., Ball, E.D., Lane, T.A.: Toxicity-evaluation designs for phase I/II cancer immunotherapy trials. Stat. Med. **29**(7–8), 712–720 (2010)

Morrissey, K.M., Yuraszeck, T.M., Li, C.-C., Zhang, Y., Kasichayanula, S.: Immunotherapy and novel combinations in oncology: current landscape, challenges, and opportunities. Clin. Transl. Sci. **9**(2), 89–104 (2016)

Thall, P., Cook, J.: Dose-finding based on efficacy-toxicity trade-offs. Biometrics **60**(3), 684–693 (2004)

Thall, P.F., Nguyen, H.Q., Braun. T.M., Qazilbash, M.H.: Using joint utlilities of the times to response and toxicity to adaptively optimize schedule-dose regimes. Biometrics **69**(3), 673–682 (2013)

Thall, P.F., Nguyen, H.Q., Zohar, S., Maton, P.: Optimizing sedative dose in preterm infants undergoing treatment for respiratory distress syndrome. J. Am. Stat. Assoc. **109**(507), 931–943 (2014)

Wang, C., Rosner, G.L., Roden, R.B.S.: A Bayesian design for phase I cancer therapeutic vaccine trials. (2018). https://doi.org/10.1002/sim.8021

Yuan, Y., Nguyen, H., Thall, P.: Bayesian Designs for Phase I-II Clinical Trials. Chapman & Hall/CRC Press, Boca Raton, FL (2016)

Printed in the United States
By Bookmasters